Unexpected Gifts

Tom Toftey

A book of nonfiction

What authors are saying

"Tom Toftey's book, Unexpected Gifts, is a wonderful story about an unexpected friendship, and how a thousand small things make for one big life. It shows us that death – even in its ugly cruelty – can open our eyes to beauty, and our hearts to generosity and love. Our friends and family will someday leave us, sure. Or we'll leave them. But if we pick up the phone, if we make a visit, we can be together today. And if love has anything to do with it, we may always be."
- David Allan Cates, author of *Tom Connor's Gift* and *Hunger in America*

"With remarkable compassion and skill, Tom Toftey shares the story of a found friendship that evolves into a profound journey through terminal illness to the very edge of life, illuminating gains and losses and above all, bestowing gifts of grace upon both the living and departed."
- John Galligan, author of nine critically acclaimed novels, including *Red Sky, Red Dragonfly, The Nail Knot,* and *Bad Axe County.*

"An ordinary summer's day on a golf course. So begins a powerful story of a man's unexpected journey to life's end and the friend who walked beside him. Although as a mystery novelist, I admire the writer for the book's 'can't put it down' quality, as a member of the human family, I applaud the story's message. I hope that others traveling a similar road may experience the love and legacy of such a friendship."
- Julie Kendrick, editor, author of *A Fatal Development* and *A Grave Matter*

"Toftey's book handles a difficult subject – the impending death of a friend – deftly and without flinching. It is a story of friendship evolving under unexpected circumstances as well as a story of surprising gifts. Toftey brings a journalist's eye and a whole lot of heart to a search for meaning and closure."
- Rod Vick, award-winning author of *Kaylee's Choice* and *The Book of Invasions*

"In Unexpected Gifts," writer Tom Toftey tells the moving story of a friendship that grew during a fatal illness. Anyone who has watched a family member move through a life-threatening disease knows how rare a friend Tom is – brave and loyal enough to keep showing up. Toftey's first book is an inspiring and ultimately life-affirming tale, one not to be missed."
- Lynette Lamb, author of *Strokeland, a Memoir: My Husband's Midlife Brainstorm and its Ambivalent Aftermath.*

"Tom Toftey's account of his visits with a dying friend brims with emotional authenticity and human goodness. While some may have drifted away from a man with little time left to live, Tom moved closer and shared the pure essence of love. This is a brief book that is chock-full of wisdom on how we might confront our own mortality with grace."
- Jess Wright, award-winning author of *A Stream to Follow*

"Sincere, sentimental, and skillful. Readers of this short, easily digestible book will witness the creation of an intimate relationship, one where death has created life rather than the reverse. Over twelve months, Toftey becomes a companion on a journey with a terminally ill man, his saintly wife, and young son. While death signals the end of life, relationships live on, and love is a rational act. A wide audience will embrace this book."

- Mike Magee, MD, medical historian, and author of **CODE BLUE:** *Inside America's Medical Industrial Complex*

"Tom Toftey's story is about discovering the art of living fully while dying. Tim becomes Tom's teacher on coping and hoping, affirming loving bonds with family and friends, and approaching death courageously. Together they reveal the power of love in the journey of living and dying well."

- Catherine Marienau, PhD, author in adult development and affective neuroscience, and a trained advocate for end-of-life options

"Poignant and inspiring, this book defines what love and friendship are. In passing from life to death, perhaps we most yearn to know that we are meaningful. This book is a loving tribute to such a life and a testament of the power that faith and friendship can provide to those around us and ultimately to ourselves."

- Craig Huegel, PhD, author of *The Nature of Plants: An Introduction to How Plants Work* and other popular ecological books

"Death happens, but dying is a process experienced only by the lucky. As Tim Hartwell's life flashed before his eyes, author Tom Toftey was able to capture each moment which grew into an unexpected gift for those Tim left behind. This story is gripping. It captured me from the moment I began reading and pulled my heartstrings throughout. While it can be read in an afternoon, its gift will last beyond a lifetime. The book will have a wide appeal, and book clubs will love it."

- Amy Ledoux, author and founder of Turtle Shell Books

Unexpected Gifts

This is a work of nonfiction.
Pseudonyms and have been used for select characters
and fictional names for some locations

Manufactured in the United States of America

ISBN: **9798874033590**

Introduction

Tim Hartwell was a loving husband, devoted father, sports enthusiast, and so much more in the prime of his life. Suddenly, on a favorite Wisconsin golf course, his life tumbled into turmoil.

I hadn't known Tim well, although years ago we had worked in the same building. I never visited his office. I didn't know his friends. We never went out for a drink after work or played a round of golf. But his call on my cellphone changed my life.

Yellow day lilies and catmint were in full bloom. So was the COVID pandemic. Our story begins in the summer warmth of 2021.

This is Tim's story. It is my story. It is our story.

But this is not the complete story of Tim's life; I couldn't begin to tell that. This is not the full story of Tim's tragedy. This book represents just a shadow of his rich life and only a hint of what he meant to others, what experiences he relished, what he had to endure.

Through my visits with Tim, we grew from being acquaintances to friends then to close friends – and the friendship we embraced through his final months was a precious, unexpected gift.

1

Wednesday, August 24, 2021

Tim teed up his ball and looked over the par five 14th hole. "*A birdie awaits,*" he thought. *Ha! Fat chance!* The narrow green 489 yards away was guarded by a creek in the front.

Methodically, he prepared to tee off. *Move the tee up a bit. Check your stance and grip. Focus. Breathe. Remember to breathe!* His routine before teeing off never changed.

But after careful preparation, he shanked his drive to the far right into the thick rough. He wasn't sure where the ball had landed, and since he played alone, he had to find it. He hated to lose even one Titleist.

"What was that shot?!" he muttered aloud, using his club to locate his ball. He recovered, but finished 14 with a triple bogey.

As he walked to 15, he reminded himself to relax, to enjoy the beauty of the day in Lake Geneva.

Geneva National, with its three courses designed by Arnold Palmer, Gary Player, and Lee Trevino, was one of Tim's favorites. He always played the Gary Player course. *"High risk, high reward,"* the golf course website said.

His tee shot from 15 was a beauty, missing the sand trap on the left of the green, giving him a chance to birdie the par three. But a near-miss putt left him with a par. He smiled contentedly. *A par's fine. A par's great!*

Tim approached 16, another par five, overlooking beautiful Lake Como. *Check your stance. Now, focus.* He sliced the ball far to the right again, missing the spacious fairway.

Not again! What is going on?

The final two holes were equally disastrous. His tee shots were off the mark; even his putts were pathetic. Tim was normally even-tempered, but he now became increasingly angry, agitated. After finishing his round, he walked quickly into the pro shop, approaching the employee at the desk.

"I just had a really bad round. No clue what is going on. Mind if I hit a few more balls?" he asked the attendant.

The attendant's face was contorted.
"I'm sorry, sir. I didn't understand anything you just said."

Tim tried again, getting out the words "some more swings," which the attendant understood.

"Yes, of course, sir."

***

Tim called his wife, Serena, who was in their room at The Ridge Hotel to let her know he had finished his round and was just hitting a few more balls. He didn't mention his erratic play. He didn't mention the attendant's confusion when he spoke. Serena wasn't at all surprised that he wanted to play a bit more. After 13 years of marriage, she was well aware of his passion for the game.

By early afternoon the Hartwell family, including 10-year-old Liam, was enjoying the warmth of an August afternoon on Williams Bay Beach. Their eight-year-old German shepherd, Sammie, was dozing on the hotel room floor.

They had looked forward to this vacation since early June when school ended. They loved The Ridge with its swimming pool and Deck Bar facing Lake Como – always a beehive of activity. Liam couldn't wait to go swimming in the clear lake near their hotel. COVID was still a concern, but they wore masks indoors most of the time. So far, they had escaped testing positive.

Serena was relieved to have some time alone, watching father and son frolic in the warm water. remembering when Liam was a newborn, spending his first nights in their home. Tim couldn't sleep. He just kept getting out of bed to look at his baby boy.

Without warning, Serena frowned, thinking about an intense conversation she had had with her boss earlier in the day. Tears flowed. Quickly, she turned so that Liam and Tim wouldn't see her crying. *What made her think about this during such a fun time with her husband and son?*

Liam loved spending time with his dad. He giggled when his dad lifted him in the water, throwing him as far as he could. He started laughing as the two of them performed underwater somersaults and handstands. When Tim carried Liam on his shoulders, Liam felt on top of the world. School begins in a few weeks. Fifth grade. He didn't want to think about it.

Thursday, August 5

Tim returned to the golf course early. He again played alone, enjoying the early morning breeze. Birds chirped from their perches in the spruce trees. A curious squirrel scooted behind a nearby shrub. A lone seagull circled overhead. *What's the gull doing here? Lake Michigan must be 30 miles away.*

His tee shots were straight; some were longer than normal. He chose his clubs carefully, wiping the dirt and grass from them so his shots would be clean. Sure, he missed some easy putts and tallied too many bogeys, but he also made a slew of pars. At least, he hadn't hit a crazy tee shot in this round!

He drove back to the hotel, jubilant, eager to tell Serena and Liam about his amazing round.

Grinning, he showed them his scorecard – a 91. The finest round of golf in his life!

"Serena, I really think I'd like to get my scorecard framed," Tim smiled. "It's a big deal."

Liam was happy for his dad, but he was even more excited to tell Tim about the miniature golf game he and his mom had played that morning. Both had made a hole-in-one.

Next on the agenda: Serena had planned a drive-through Wisconsin wildlife safari for the afternoon. While she drove, Liam sat in front, allowing him to spot the animals. Tim was unusually quiet in the back seat. Serena assumed he was tired from his early morning tee time. Perhaps he was just replaying his landmark round of golf in his mind.

They drove to Chuck's Lakeshore Inn in nearby Fontana for supper. Liam was always hungry. Tim volunteered to take their orders to the outdoor bar. Without hesitation, Liam opted for a burger with lettuce and ketchup. When Serena requested a chicken Caesar salad, Tim looked confused. He just stood there, as if he had never heard of a chicken Caesar salad.

Almost sarcastically, Serena repeated her order very deliberately.

"Tim! Tim? I'd like a c-h-i-c-k-e-n C-a-es-a-r s-a-l-a-d."

He didn't reply; he just walked to the bar to place their order.

2

Friday, August 6

Knowing the golf course was busy on a Friday, Tim decided to spend the day with Serena and Liam. Liam wanted to go to the Lake Geneva Pie Company for breakfast. Serena and Tim voted to get breakfast to-go from Joni's Diner, then take it to the Pie Company to eat outside. Liam grinned when his mom handed him a generous slice of apple pie from the Pie Company.

Around noon, Tim drove them back to the golf course. He wanted to buy a memento in celebration of his fantastic round of golf. After parking and turning off the engine, Tim looked at Serena, trying to speak, but all that came out was "rrr-rrrr-rr-rrr."

"Stop! Stop!" Serena cried. "What are you saying? Tim, tell me again!"

Tim looked confused. *Why can't I pronounce the words I want to say?* It was like his brain was stuck. Like an old record skipping.

"Are you okay?" Serena asked.

"Yeah."

Tim got out of the car. His shoulders sagged. He looked defeated. Instead of walking toward the golf shop, he paced around the parking lot. Serena and Liam watched, bewildered.

"What's Dad doing, Mom?" Liam asked from the back seat.

"Are you okay?" Serena screamed. "You're scaring me." She felt panicky as she got out of the car, taking his hands in hers. They weren't clammy as she had suspected. She didn't feel any weakness in his hands, but he didn't look at her.

"Yeah. I'm fine. I'm fine." He spoke slowly, but clearly. He walked some more, in denial that anything was wrong.

Serena watched Tim walk toward the golf pro shop. He seemed to be walking just fine. Nonetheless, she worried. She whispered to Liam asking him to catch up to his dad. She wanted to FaceTime with him, to hear Tim speak, to be sure that he was okay. As Liam walked beside his dad, Serena searched the internet for the nearest emergency room.

While Tim paid the pro shop attendant for a long-sleeve fleece pull-over, Liam moved behind a rack of sport shirts to FaceTime, "Mom, he was saying some wrong words – 'wind' instead of 'window' and 'flow' instead of 'floor.'"

Serena had moved to the driver's seat. As Tim got in beside her, Serena sighed nervously.

"Something isn't right, Tim. Should we go to the ER?"

"No. I'm okay," he protested. Serena wasn't so sure.

"Maybe we should go back to the hotel to rest a little," Serena suggested. "We've had a busy morning."

"Yeah, that would be okay," Tim replied, thinking he might be dehydrated.

When they opened their hotel room door, Sammie was waiting, wagging his tail then licking Liam's hand. Tim was relieved to lie on the bed. A glass of water quenched his thirst. The washcloth on his forehead felt soothing. His eyes were focused. He squeezed Serena's hands smiling a little.

"Tim, let's talk a little," Serena said. She proceeded to ask him several questions: What is the date of Liam's birthday? When did we get married? What is the name of our hotel? Tim answered each question correctly, but some of his speech was slurred.

Tim tried to speak, but only uttered gibberish. Liam looked at his mom, confused and worried.

"I don't want to scare you, Tim, but I'm taking you to the ER."

Without saying a word, Tim rose from the bed, then shuffled into the bathroom. Serena and Liam heard him vigorously brushing his teeth. Then, silence. They looked at each other, waiting. Then they heard Tim begin to cry, softly at first, then sobbing. Serena whispered to Liam, "Dad hasn't cried since Grandma died."

"Oh, something's wrong!" Tim yelled while stumbling from the bathroom. "Something's wrong! Get me some help!" His terrified look frightened Liam, but he steadied his dad, as Tim put his arm around his son's shoulders.

Serena quickly called the hotel's front desk, frantically asking the staff member to call 911 to take her husband to the nearest ER. Tim seemed to be unaware of what was happening. Liam helped him sit. Sammie moved to the far corner of the room.

Serena sat beside Tim, trying to reassure him that the ambulance would arrive soon. Tim didn't understand her.

"Why aren't you taking me?" Tim cried aloud. "I need help! Something's wrong!"

"An ambulance is on its way, Tim," Serena assured him, sitting beside him, holding his hands, calming him.

***

As the EMTs lifted Tim into the ambulance, he was conscious but unable to speak. Sirens wailed during the half-hour drive to Mercyhealth Hospital and Medical Center in nearby Walworth.

Serena and Tim had driven to Lake Geneva separately, since Tim wanted to stop enroute to visit his 91-year-old father. She opted to drive her car to Mercyhealth. Before leaving, Serena stopped at the front desk, to alert the staff what was happening. The woman was empathetic and helpful, offering to help with their dog, Sammie. Serena was grateful.

As soon as the ambulance arrived, ER staff gave Tim a CT scan which ruled out a stroke. A second scan with contrast was administered. The doctor informed Serena that his second scan showed a suspicious area on his brain.

Serena couldn't breathe. *What had he just said? Something about Tim's brain?*

"We're not equipped to handle this here," the doctor said. "Your husband needs a higher level of care." Liam remained silent, then watched his mother reach for her cellphone.

Serena acted quickly. She called Shaun O'Leary, a respected neurosurgeon in Chicagoland. More importantly, he was Tim's friend and golf buddy. He and Tim had been colleagues at Evanston Northwestern Healthcare ten years earlier.

Shaun suggested Lutheran General Hospital in Park Ridge where he had privileges, as the next step for Tim. After calling the hospital, Shaun told Serena that Tim couldn't be transferred until evening when a bed became available.

For more than four hours, Serena and Liam waited with Tim in the ER at Mercyhealth. Tim was confused, unable to process what was happening. He fell asleep then awoke with a start. Occasionally, he spoke to Serena. Liam listened, watching his dad, while observing the nurses as they scurried around. He giggled a little hearing Tim's nonsensical language, wondering whether his dad was just being silly. "Liam, he can't help that. It's not really funny," Serena whispered.

Serena was frightened, trying to organize her thoughts. She needed to stay with Tim. She needed to console Liam. She needed to pack their belongings into the cars. She needed to fetch Sammie from the hotel room then check out of the hotel. She needed to figure how to get Tim's car back home. Serena was overwhelmed. Mother and son held hands as they waited.

When the ambulance arrived, Tim didn't understand what was happening. Serena looked into Tim's eyes, seeing only confusion. That broke her heart.

"You'll be okay, Tim," Serena said, touching his hand. "The doctors will take care of you." Serena and Liam returned to the hotel. Liam helped his mom with everything, making several trips back and forth, packing both cars with suitcases and other belongings. *What would she have done without Liam?* She took the key to Tim's car to the front desk. She would ask a friend to get the car later. As she and Liam pulled out of the parking lot, a gentle rain began.

Near the Illinois border, a nurse from Lutheran General Hospital called Serena, inquiring about Tim's medical history. She called her parents to tell them Tim was being hospitalized. Next, she contacted his brother, Phil, who promised to meet the ambulance at the hospital. Serena was relieved. Her head was spinning. The rain was falling harder now. *Keep your eyes on the road. Just 40 miles to go.*

In a steady rain, Serena drove Liam and Sammie back to their home in northwest Chicago, arriving around 11 p.m. She needed to stay with Liam. They were drained, physically and emotionally, as they unpacked the car. She noticed a neighbor's light was on, and quickly stopped to tell her what was happening. While Serena unlocked her door, she suspected another neighbor could hear her sobbing through an open window.

Although it was very late, she called the parents of one of Liam's friends, asking them to care for him on Saturday. She phoned another friend who offered to host Liam on Sunday. *Thank God, Liam has tennis camp for a week beginning Monday. That will allow me to be with Tim.*

***

Saturday, August 7

Serena and Tim's brother met with a neurosurgeon in the ICU on Saturday morning. He told them that Tim's MRI, conducted after midnight, had identified a tumor. "The MRI shows a circle with two prongs," the physician said. *"What does that mean?"* Serena wondered.

"A biopsy of Tim's brain has been scheduled for early Monday," he said, interrupting her thoughts. "The pathology report can take up to five days."

Sitting beside Tim, Serena remained quiet, letting him rest. Tim's peripheral vision was affected, so he couldn't see her, but he sensed her nearby. Serena felt frightened, alone. She reached for Tim's hand, stroking it, wondering how she would cope.

At home that night, Serena told Liam that something was very wrong with his dad. Liam looked at her, with a sad, worried expression on his face. Liam knew that his dad's language had been affected. She didn't want her son to worry, but of course, he did. They both worried.

***

Sunday, August 8

Serena spent the day in Tim's room. Minors weren't allowed in the ICU, so she was grateful her friend was caring for Liam. A neighbor offered to take Sammie on walks.

Tim remained confused throughout the day. That afternoon, a speech therapist came to visit him. Serena was frightened when she observed them talking. Tim wasn't able to name any colors, not even one. The therapist didn't prolong her visit.

Serena wasn't hungry. In time, she'd eat an apple or granola bar she had poked into her purse before leaving home. Her mind was a blur. She couldn't call anyone. She couldn't cry. A thoughtful nurse gave Serena a pillow and blanket. She couldn't sleep, but she rested, trying to remain calm. Tim drifted in and out of sleep.

At one point, Serena got up. She thought she had heard Tim say something, but he was asleep.

She sat beside him, massaging his arm then kissing his hand. *Tim, I wish I could help you.*

She left the hospital, weary, feeling empty. She hardly remembered leaving the parking lot to pick up Liam at their friends' home. She was eager to hug Liam.

3

Monday, August 9

After walking with Liam to the nearby tennis camp, Serena returned to Lutheran General, anxious to see Tim. She sat in his room, feeling isolated as she waited for Tim to return following his brain biopsy. Minutes of waiting. Then hours. Time to think. *Perhaps Tim's tumor is benign. Perhaps he will be okay. Perhaps. Perhaps.*

As Tim was wheeled to his room, Serena noticed how very quiet the nurse was. She didn't speak to Serena. The silence was eerie. Serena stood beside Tim, tenderly touching his face. Tim was asleep.

Minutes later, she overheard the nurses in the hall whispering – "It's bad." Serena's heart broke. She wept quietly. Alone.

How could Tim have a brain tumor of all things? He's one of the smartest people I know. How will I manage? What should I tell Liam? Can they remove the tumor? I need to get home for Liam.

***

Tuesday, August 10

Again, Serena walked with Liam to tennis camp, then stayed with Tim at Lutheran General.

Gradually, Tim became more aware, and he looked to Serena for answers. She tried to explain what the medical staff was doing. She wasn't certain that Tim understood, but he listened intently. He trusted his wife completely. She felt strengthened by his trust, while absorbing the pressure of shouldering that trust.

Throughout the day, Tim drifted in and out of sleep.

Serena called her boss to tell her that she needed some time off to care for Tim. Her boss understood, suggesting that she take Family and Medical Leave for as long as necessary. Serena also called a colleague from her job as Director of Imaging at University of Illinois Health. She needed to confide in someone. Otherwise, communication with her colleagues and friends was limited to texting. She just didn't have the energy to talk with anyone by phone.

Neighbors and friends were wonderful. They organized a "meal train," delivering meals and goodies to Serena and Liam.

Their close friend, Shaun, phoned occasionally for updates. Although he specialized in spine surgery instead of brain surgery, his counsel was invaluable. His calm, nurturing voice bolstered Serena's spirit. He cared about his friend Tim.

While Tim rested, Serena couldn't help thinking that a week ago, Tim, Liam, and she had been in Lake Geneva, taking Sammie on a relaxing walk around the hotel property, feeling the joy of being together on vacation. She smiled remembering how much Sammie loved sniffing in an area overgrown with brush and trees near the hotel. *What a difference a week makes.*

***

Wednesday, August 11

Tim ate very little while he was in the neurology ICU. When he wanted something, Serena had to help him. He couldn't understand the words on the menu or comprehend the process of ordering food. After his breakfast arrived, he slept soundly.

A staff physician entered Tim's ICU room. Serena had so many questions, but the physician had no answers, since she hadn't had any previous contact with Tim. Serena firmly asked the nursing staff never to have this staff physician return. The nurses honored her request.

Finally, Tim's neurosurgeon met with Serena and Tim. He smiled briefly, then became serious as he sat beside Serena.

"The pathology results from the biopsy show that Tim has Stage 4 brain cancer – Glioblastoma Multiforme (GBM). This is the most aggressive of all brain cancers. I'm so sorry, Tim and Serena." Serena couldn't speak. She felt weak. Tim was somber as he struggled to comprehend.

"Tim needs to have surgery soon," the neurosurgeon continued. "We'll make arrangements here at Lutheran General."

Serena told the doctor she would talk this over with their good friend, neurosurgeon Shaun O'Leary. When Shaun learned that Tim had glioblastoma, he became very quiet. *Oh no, not glioblastoma.* Clearly, he was emotional, as he offered Serena support. She told him that the neurosurgeon at Lutheran General had suggested scheduling a surgery date.

Shaun hesitated, then replied, "You know, Serena, it's not unusual to shop around for a surgeon. I know a neurosurgeon at Illinois Masonic Hospital who has experience with brain tumors affecting speech. Dr. Kenji Muro trained under me and was my colleague. He's very skilled, and Illinois Masonic is close to your home, Serena. I think Tim should be transferred there." Serena trusted Shaun. The decision was made.

***

Thursday, August 12

Visiting hours began at 9:30 a.m. at Lutheran General, but Serena arrived early, feeling impatient. She was anxious to know how Tim's night had been, when he would be released, what type of care he would need at home. The wait for answers lasted several hours.

"Take a deep breath," she thought.

Tim was released that afternoon to return home. He was quiet riding in the car. When they opened the door to their home, Sammie greeted them, wagging his tail furiously. Tim smiled as he gave his lovable dog a pat. "I missed you, Sammie," Tim whispered. Serena assisted Tim as he climbed the stairs. He paused before sitting on the sofa, obviously drained of energy.

Serena was frustrated that she had received so few instructions from hospital staff, but Tim was stable, and he was home! Serena looked over at Tim from the kitchen, relieved to see him sitting on the couch, scratching Sammie behind his ears. *They are such pals.*

When Liam returned from tennis camp, he grinned, thrilled to see his dad again. He walked toward him, not quite daring to hug him. Six days had passed since he last saw his dad, but he felt awkward, not knowing what to say or do. He wondered whether he would understand his dad. He remained quiet, as he walked into the kitchen to get a snack.

4

Friday, August 13

The neurosurgeon, Dr. Kenji Muro, arrived in jeans for the meeting with Tim and Serena at Illinois Masonic, a six-minute drive from the Hartwell home. Perhaps, he had interrupted his day off as a favor to their mutual friend Shaun. Dr. Muro's personable nature was evident as he spoke to them. Direct. Thorough. Empathetic.

Imaging scans had been sent to him from Lutheran General. Dr. Muro reviewed the MRI with them both. He looked at Serena and Tim with the eyes of wisdom from his experience as a neurosurgeon, but also as a sensitive, caring human being.

"What questions do you have?" Dr. Muro asked.

"How long do I have?" Tim spoke immediately. His speech was understandable.

"Looking at the MRI, I would estimate that you will live between 12 and 14 months, Tim," Dr. Muro said. "I am so very sorry."

Bowing her head, Serena's eyes glistened with tears. Tim too was stunned, but he quickly replied, "I'm going to break that record." Dr. Muro and Serena exchanged glances, surprised by Tim's positivity.

"Tim's surgery to remove the tumor has been scheduled for September 9," Dr. Muro said. *"September 9 can't come quickly enough,"* Serena thought.

On August 14, Tim's father and brother visited. He was happy to see them. This may have been difficult for his dad, but everyone tried to keep the mood light. They ordered pizza to lift their spirits. Liam was pleased! They all were.

***

During the next several days, Serena contacted relatives and a few colleagues, while his brother called some of Tim's high school pals. Tim talked with his siblings, encouraging them to call him frequently. He was eager to hear stories about their parents and his childhood.

Two of Tim's closest friends, Scott Dickson and Drew Nielsen, were stunned when they heard the news of Tim's diagnosis. Scott lived in California and Drew lived in Florida, but the three of them had a special bond that spanned decades.

***

On August 20, Serena and Tim took a walk on Montrose Beach. They loved breathing the fresh air, watching the gentle waves of Lake Michigan lap against the shore. They carried their shoes as they waded in the warm water.

It had been nine days since Tim's diagnosis. Surgery hadn't yet taken place. Treatments hadn't begun. Serena wished time could stand still; she feared it would run out all too soon.

After receiving Tim's bleak diagnosis, they understood that his disease was terminal. As they strolled, Tim took Serena's hand, looked at Serena and said, "After I die, I want to come back as a seagull."

"Don't you think seagulls are dirty and annoying?" Serena asked.

"No. They get to soar through the air, flying freely, eating snacks."

Serena agreed. That made sense.

"Which shoulder do you want me to land on?" Tim wondered.

"The left, because you are left-handed," Serena replied, stifling a smile.

They walked a while in silence, pausing to look as far as they could across Lake Michigan. Serena marveled at how they were talking about this so casually.

5

I usually take a daily walk with my dog, Digger, in the forest preserve in my hometown of Winfield, Illinois, past the burial grounds of Native Americans, onto a shaded forest path.

But today, August 15, 2021, I am walking alone through our neighborhood, past nicely groomed lawns, attractive homes and colorful flower beds. Birds sing from their perches. A pair of ducks float lazily in a small pond along my route.

I walk near a parochial school, noticing a young woman exiting her Toyota.

"Excuse me," I begin. "It's summer vacation. I'm surprised to see any cars in the school parking lot this early."

"Oh, a few staff members have jobs throughout the summer," she said, "and some of us are getting our rooms ready for the first days of school."

As I wish her well, passing the school's wildflower garden, my phone rings, but I don't recognize the number. *Probably a nuisance call.* Then, I notice the 773-area code. Chicago. *I'd better answer.*

"Hi Tom. This is Tim Hartwell. I have some bad news. I just found out I have stage four brain cancer, and it's the worst kind."

No preliminaries. Just brutal honesty.

I was surprised to hear from Tim; we hadn't talked in many months. We had been colleagues at the American Medical Association in Chicago for several years, but we weren't close. We worked in different departments, on different floors in the AMA's 17-floor building.

I didn't have a chance to reply, before Tim launched: He told me about golfing in Lake Geneva, having difficulty speaking to the golf pro, swimming with his son, crying in the bathroom, seeing his wife worry, being taken to a Chicago hospital. He talked quickly, grasping for the right words. His speech was a bit off. "I was playing the best golf of my life," Tim said, "and then I started muffing the ball."

"Can you understand me, Tom? I know I don't speak right sometimes."

"Yes, I can understand you, Tim. I am so sorry you're going through this. Stage four cancer – that's awful. How can I help you?"

Tim didn't answer. I wasn't sure whether he understood me. "Would you like me to visit you sometime, Tim?" I asked.

"Oh, that would be great," he said, before saying goodbye.

***

Tim Hartwell. I remembered him as a handsome, friendly guy with a warm smile and a passion for sports, especially baseball and golf. Our jobs at the AMA didn't overlap; I didn't even know where he worked within the AMA. As far as I knew, we didn't have mutual friends. We met because we both enjoyed entering low-stakes sports pools among our colleagues – predicting college bowl games, March Madness, NFL games and major golf tournaments.

We occasionally ran into each other in the AMA lobby where we'd chat about a game. One day, I spotted him sitting alone in the AMA cafeteria, so I joined him. That turned into occasional lunches together. He was an ardent Chicago Bears fan; I maintained my Viking allegiance after growing up in Minnesota. He supported his alma mater, Purdue University; I cheered for the Wisconsin Badgers having earned my master's degree at the UW. We shared one favorite team though – the Chicago Cubs. Tim was a Cubs loyalist; my interest was more episodic, except when the Cubs made a run in the National League.

Our lunches in the AMA cafeteria became routine. We enjoyed each other's company. We shared travel experiences, discussed childhood adventures and family information. When one of our sports pools was approaching, we'd compare notes and strategies.

In 2002, Tim left the AMA for a job at Evanston Northwestern Healthcare where he became a practice manager in the division of neurosurgery. After working at the AMA for 22 years, I retired a year later, ready to venture into the world of consulting. Our communication faded, except in telephone conversations after entering a sports pool, either celebrating our wins or commiserating over dismal finishes in the pools. Tim did better in the weekly NFL pools; I had some success in the four major golf tournament pools – the Masters, PGA Championship, US Open and the British Open.

The driving distance between my home and Chicago and the busyness of our lives hindered getting together, but in 2008, I attended Tim and Serena's beautiful wedding on the North Side of Chicago at Salvatore's. I knew very few people at the wedding.

We exchanged Christmas cards every year, and I was delighted to receive a baby photo of Liam in October 2010. Tim's message on the card reflected the immense joy he felt in being a dad.

6

On Monday, August 23, 2021, I visited Tim for the first time since his call. It took me an hour to drive from Winfield to Tim's home in northwest Chicago, a part of the city that was unfamiliar to me.

Because COVID continued to be frightening, my wife, Jane, and I hadn't ventured into Chicago in a long time, so making the drive into the city was daunting, but I felt visiting Tim was important. I knew Tim and his family would be wearing masks.

Jane and I typically wore masks while maintaining social distance outside our home. We were especially careful, because Jane has a chronic disease called sarcoidosis of the lungs and lymph nodes. There is no cure. Testing positive for COVID could be disastrous for her. Nonetheless, Jane understood my need to visit Tim.

Tim's home was on a quiet street. I worried that finding a parking place on the street would be difficult, but it wasn't. The townhouse was in an attractive brick complex with a courtyard filled with colorful flowers, trees, and outdoor patios separated by wrought iron fences. No one was outside when I arrived. Evidently, residents were at work in the city or more likely on Zoom in their homes, due to COVID restrictions.

After ringing the doorbell, I put on my mask and waited a brief time until Tim opened the door. His eyes radiated pleasure above his mask. Inside the lower entryway, I met Sammie, his lovable German shepherd. Sammie and I became friends. Tim told me that Sammie preferred spending much of his time during the summer months in his dog bed on the cool lower floor.

I followed Tim up the stairs to the main living area. He walked slowly, carefully. At the top of the stairway was a dining table, spacious living room, bathroom and kitchen. Serena greeted me warmly, but her face reflected the worry and stress she had endured for the past several weeks. I had last seen her as Tim's beautiful bride thirteen years earlier. She suggested that Tim and I visit in the living room.

Tim sat on the sofa. The coffee table in front of him was cluttered with books, notes, magazines, a calendar, and post-it reminders. Around the room were several bookcases, a large television, photos, and artistic touches everywhere.

This must be where Tim spends his days.

Settling into a comfortable chair facing Tim, I told him how happy I was to see him looking so well. Indeed, he did. He was trim and appeared healthy, much like our days together at the AMA.

   Without preliminaries, Tim catapulted into a monologue, recapping his golfing days in Lake Geneva, the best golf score he had ever had, then the slices from the tees which were the worst he had experienced. I let him talk. He told me about how angry he was with his shanks far off the fairway, how he asked the golf attendant to play a bit longer. Then, he told me that the attendant didn't understand him.
His speech was labored as he struggled to find the right words. I tried my best to interpret what he was saying; I didn't correct him. For the most part, I understood the gist of his story.

When he began repeating the golf story, I asked a few questions to divert him: Were Serena and Liam with you? How old is Liam now? Did you like your hotel? Did you find any great restaurants in Lake Geneva? Do Serena and Liam play golf too?

These questions seemed to give him a break from dwelling on what happened. He described how beautiful the Gary Player course was, how much he loved being in the fresh air, how pleased he was to be playing alone.

Then, Tim shifted gears, away from the golf course to his family. He was so grateful that Serena and Liam were with him in Lake Geneva when he had become disoriented. He talked about how all of them looked forward to taking their vacation in this beautiful part of southern Wisconsin. He recalled how much fun it was to go swimming with his son.

"Liam really hasn't fallen in love with golf yet, but some day he might," he said. "I'm going to encourage him to take golf lessons. You really need lessons when you're starting out. I sure hope Liam and I will be able to play some golf together." Tim's voice faded as he spoke. Thinking. Imagining. Wondering.

We both remained quiet. I was about to ask Tim a question when he interrupted me.

"Do you want to see our roof deck?" he asked.
"That'd be great."

We walked up a flight of stairs to the third level, and then another flight to get to the roof. He wasn't as winded as I thought he might be after climbing the stairs. He smiled broadly as he showed me the roof deck. Comfortable deck furniture and plants gave the deck a cozy feeling. The view overlooking the courtyard below and buildings in the distance was wonderful. As he sat in one of the chairs, he suggested that we talk there for a while. The summer breeze felt refreshing. Our conversation drifted from one topic to another.

"My cancer is really bad, Tom – the worst kind," he said, "but I'm not in pain. I feel pretty good. I just get tired a lot."

"That's understandable," I replied. "Your fatigue must be tough. This just isn't fair."

"Really, I'm so lucky, Tom," Tim said. "Lucky that Serena is such a wonderful wife. Lucky to have such a smart son. Lucky to own the best dog in the whole world."

A lump formed in my throat, and tears rested in my eyes. *He's terminally ill – and he feels lucky. Incredible.*

I was amazed how clearly he spoke sometimes, then how quickly his speech became incoherent. I had to listen closely to decipher what he was trying to say.

"I'm having surgery in two or three weeks," Tim announced. "I don't know what that will be like. Maybe it will tell me more about how bad my cancer is. I know it's bad," he said, "but I hope to live a long time." He became quiet.

"Tim, is it okay if I contact Rob Camin and Tom Conway from your days at the AMA?" I asked. "I think they would like to know about you."

"Sure. That would be great. I want people to know about my brain cancer," he replied. "When I called you, I called some other people too but not those guys. Serena helped me make a list."

"Have you kept in touch with Tom and Rob?"

"No, not really. I don't think I stayed close to any of the staff at the AMA," he said.

Finally, he stood up, motioning me to join him at the railing overlooking the courtyard.

***

"I hope to get a really good telescope someday," he said. He struggled with that word "telescope," but I understood.

"This would be a great place to use a scope," he suggested. "I hope Liam will like using it. We had one when I was young. It was complicated, but I loved looking through it."

His eyes drifted away, lost in thought. *Perhaps, he's thinking back to his childhood, imagining something.* He remained motionless, focusing on the courtyard below for a long time. Then his eyes moved slowly upward to the blue sky. My eyes followed his.

"I don't know when I will die, maybe in three months – or three years. When I am gone, maybe Serena and Liam will come up here some night to look through the telescope – to look at the stars. Maybe they will think of me. Perhaps they will talk to me." Tim stood still.

I couldn't move. I couldn't speak. My eyes glistened as I put my hand on his shoulder. We just stood together for a long time, looking at the heavens, feeling a slight breeze on our faces.

As we walked downstairs, I could tell that Tim was tiring. I told him that I needed to head home but would call him soon.

"That would be great, Tom. Thanks for coming," he said, smiling.

Serena walked with me downstairs so that she could lock the door after I left.

"Tim tires easily," Serena said.

"Did I stay too long, Serena?" I asked.

"No. I could tell he loved talking with you," she replied. "He hasn't had many visitors. Were you able to understand him?"

"Yes, for the most part. A few times I wasn't sure what he was saying, but I didn't want to interrupt him to ask. I was afraid to embarrass him."

"Liam and I do the same thing, but sometimes I can tell he really wants to say the right word, so I correct him. I often write words for him because that seems to help." *Serena and Liam have to be very patient as Tim speaks.*

I asked her when Tim's surgery would take place. She knew the date without checking: September 9 – in 17 days. I asked how long Tim would be in the hospital after surgery, but she wasn't sure. She offered to text me to let me know how the surgery went. I hugged her gently, hoping that Serena would feel my support and empathy.

I drove home that day, thinking of Tim and how he was coping. I thought of Serena and how her life had changed since that Friday in Lake Geneva. I thought of young Liam, imagining how confused he must be.

My mind returned to the roof deck where we stood at the railing looking at the courtyard below then at the heavens above. Tim treasured that silence. He was teaching me the value of relishing the quiet moments in life, the time to reflect without words.

When I arrived home, Jane asked me how my visit with Tim had been. I started to tell her about Tim's memorable words, "I am so lucky." I lost it. I started crying.

Reflecting on my first visit, I realized that Tim might continue to replay his experience on the Geneva National Golf Course whenever I visited. While this might be important for him to retell his experience now and then, I decided to prepare for my next visit by writing a list of questions to keep our conversation stimulating.

7

My current career prepared me well for future visits with Tim. After leaving the AMA in March 2003, I became a communications consultant, ready to work for clients needing help in public relations, corporate relations, or marketing.

I often telephoned my elderly mother during those days since she was in her mid-90s, living in a care center in my hometown of Grand Marais, Minnesota. She was always interested in what was happening with Jane and me, so I called to tell her that I had retired early from the AMA and had started a consulting company.

"Oh, are you sure you should have done that?" she asked. She said the same thing when I left my first career in teaching high school English and journalism at Memorial High School in Madison, Wisconsin, after 11 years.

"Yes, I've always wanted to try my hand in owning a consulting company," I said.

"How many people are in your company?" Mom was still fairly sharp. There was nothing wrong with her hearing. In fact, nurses at the care center told me that she occasionally corrected their grammar from across the dining room.

"Just me," I said.

"Oh," perhaps a bit disappointed. "What's the name of your company?" she asked.

"Toftey Consulting."

"Not very creative." At 95, my mother was still alert. In my first year as a consultant, I landed a number of clients including a medical specialty, biotech company, medical awards organization, and small foundation.

A call from a pharmaceutical company changed the trajectory in that first year of Toftey Consulting. My contact at Astra Zeneca Pharmaceuticals, Steve, had heard that I was retiring early from the AMA, and he asked to meet me at O'Hare Airport. He and a colleague were flying to Chicago in a week. Steve hoped to hire me as a consultant, suggesting that I meet them in a conference room at the United Club with a one-page bulleted list of what I thought I could do for Astra Zeneca.

An empty sheet of lined paper sat on my office desk for several days. Although I had visited numerous pharmaceutical, biotech, and medical device companies in my role as Corporate Relations Director for the AMA, I had never worked for one. But eventually, I thought of one idea. And then another. By the time I drove to O'Hare to meet Steve and his colleague, I had filled a page with ideas.

When I gave my list to the Astra Zeneca folks, they quietly studied it, without saying a word, without telegraphing their reaction.

"Well, I blew that one," I thought.

They looked at each other, and Steve smiled. "We need every one of your ideas, Tom."

I was hired to work about 25-30 hours per month. The work was fascinating. I traveled occasionally to their corporate office in Wilmington, Delaware. During my time at AZ, I interviewed all levels of employees for a project. That job alone paid for the wedding of our daughter, Jamie, to her husband, Patrick. But – I knew that this job would cease at the end of the calendar year, so I would need to market myself to other potential clients.

***

Another bit of good fortune occurred on a United flight from Chicago to San Francisco, when I sat next to a man whose laptop was open. I couldn't help noticing incredible photos of his home, hanging on the cliffs near San Francisco Bay, and we started talking. He asked what I did for a living; then, I asked about his job.

"I moderate focus groups for food companies," he said.

"Sounds interesting," I replied. "Tell me more." I had participated in a few focus groups but really knew very little about them. I didn't recall any of the moderators. During the four-hour flight, he described his world of qualitative research, moderating focus groups of 8-10 consumers and conducting in-depth interviews with executives, all for food companies around the country. He even shared financial details from his work as an independent moderator. I was fascinated.

"Asking questions, then probing for greater depth in respondents' answers, is the key," he told me. "The challenges are this job requires a lot of travel and qualitative research is very competitive. There are a lot of independent moderators all over the country."

When I returned to Winfield, I contacted a woman who moderated focus groups to join me for lunch and conversation, read a couple books about moderating, then attended an intense three-day seminar to learn the fine points of being a moderator. I returned home ready to embark with new skills and capabilities for Toftey Consulting.

Now, after moderating for nearly 20 years, I figured that asking Tim a variety of questions then probing for information would come naturally.

8

Serena was kind to call or text me occasionally. She was happy to tell me that Tim's childhood friend, Drew, had recently been in touch.

When Drew Nielsen received a text from Serena that Tim had the worst type of brain cancer, glioblastoma, he called Tim from his home in Florida.

Tim was delighted hearing Drew's voice, but Tim dominated the conversation.

Drew just listened, amazed at Tim's outlook in dealing with his terrible disease.

"I've been dealt a blow – but how can I complain?" Tim started. "Think of all the kids who have cancer and live for a year or two." Listening to his friend, Drew started to cry – and then, so did Tim.

In time, Tim continued, "Do you remember Lou Gehrig's famous speech?"

Drew recalled that when Gehrig was hit by ALS – amyotrophic lateral sclerosis – at age 36, he addressed the crowd at Yankee Stadium in an emotional farewell. The famous phrase from his speech, "I am the luckiest man on the face of the earth," resonated with Tim. He took it to heart.

"Guess what I just figured, Drew. I was diagnosed on the 20,000[th] day of my life! Isn't that amazing? I'm going to make the most of the time I have left," Tim said.

"That's a great attitude," Drew said, promising to fly to Chicago when he was able.

***

My opportunities to visit Tim during the fall of 2021 were limited, because I had knee replacement surgery followed by physical therapy. I settled for occasional phone conversations.

I started telling him about my knee surgery, but he was only mildly interested, so I told him about an earlier medical experience. I had awakened in the recovery room after getting my knee scoped. When I looked at the guy on the gurney next to me – there was Bo Jackson, the amazing athlete who excelled in two professional sports. Tim laughed a little – he knew Bo!

Of course, Bo was there under an assumed name, but I recognized him immediately. I teased Tim by telling him about my *lengthy* conversation with Bo:

Tom: "How are you doing?"

Bo: "Probably as well as you."

Tim smiled, chuckling a little, understanding the humor. (That surgery may have ended Bo's career in the NFL.)

He was excited to tell me that Serena had taken him to Navy Pier for a pep rally for his beloved University of Southern California football team, preparing to play Notre Dame. Serena had secretly contacted the university athletic department, mentioning Tim's illness, loyalty to USC football, and his excitement at attending the pep rally in Chicago. During the rally Tim was surprised when the athletic director called his name, then presented him with a football signed by all of the Trojan football players. He was ecstatic.

***

My time in visiting Tim during that fall was further complicated when a market research company hired me to work on a lengthy dermatology project interviewing various medical professionals via Zoom.

I kept in touch with Tim by telephone, timing my calls to when Liam was in school and Serena at her job. He always seemed pleased to hear from me. Although he alluded to his golf experience at Lake Geneva and being rushed to the hospital, he no longer dwelt on it.

Tim focused on staying positive. He decided that since he could no longer work, he would do what he enjoyed – reading magazines and books, watching golf tournaments and college football games, and viewing reruns of old major league baseball games. In one call, he reminded me how much he loved baseball when he was a kid growing up in Prosper, Illinois, a town far west of Chicago.

"I played all the time during the summer. I remember that my friend Drew and I had to sprint home sometimes with minutes to spare before supper."

"Drew called me the other day. He doesn't live around here. He really got me laughing. It felt so good to just laugh and laugh," Tim said. "He asked if I remembered our fourth-grade teacher, and I did. She had red hair. Drew agreed, then reminded me that she was a *Little House on the Prairie* fanatic." Tim had trouble pronouncing that word "fanatic," but I figured it out.

"Did you and Drew both play for the Prosper High School team?" I asked.

"No, and I was really sad," he said. "Drew decided to go to a private school instead. I didn't see him much."

"So, you lost contact?"

"Yeah, for quite a while, but one day after I finished college, I went to a park in Prosper to shoot hoops, and Drew was there," Tim answered. "We couldn't believe it. It had been so long. Then, we started playing golf together, and we've been good friends ever since."

"But I thought Drew didn't live around here," I said.

"Yeah, he moved to Florida. At least I think it's Florida, but now I'm not sure. I should ask Serena," he replied.

"Serena? Serena!" he yelled.

"Serena is at work, Tim – but that's okay," I said. "You can ask her when she gets home." I could tell that he was frustrated not knowing where his good friend lived. I could imagine that Serena likely was called upon daily to answer a flurry of questions.

***

In mid-September, Tim called me. He didn't call often, but he was eager to tell me about his brain surgery to remove the tumor. "The surgery took eight hours, and I had to be awake the whole time!" Tim exclaimed. "The pain was the worst I've experienced. My surgeon told me afterward that no other pain could be as bad as this, and that any pain before dying would be far less."

Tim told me that Serena, his brother Phil, and his dad had waited in a lounge for his surgery to end. Because of COVID restrictions, they had to confine their visits to one at a time.

Tim continued, "I told Phil that if I had known how terrible the surgery would be, I wouldn't have done it. He told me I was brave, and we both cried. After that awful pain, I told him that I was going to beat this cancer."

I couldn't imagine having to be awake during any surgery, let alone an eight-hour brain surgery.

Talking with Tim by phone was far more difficult than in person. He listened to my questions and tried, but his speech continued to be difficult to decipher. If he couldn't think of the word "lake" he might say "water" or "ocean." If he couldn't think of the words "catcher's mitt," he might say "thing," or simply use guttural sounds that made no sense. Of course, he may have thought he was pronouncing the words correctly. If he wasn't able to communicate well, he became frustrated trying so hard to say the words he wanted. Even over the phone, I could sense his torment.

In another call, he wanted to talk about the Cubs because they were on a nice string of wins.

"Did you get to any of the Cubs' World Series games?" he asked.

"No – tickets were too hard to get," I replied, "and too expensive."

He then proceeded to talk about the Cubs' landmark win in 2016, beating the Cleveland Indians for the World Series title, its first since 1908. Anthony Rizzo and Kris Bryant were among his favorite players – mine too. For whatever reason, his speech was better than normal that day. We both laughed when we realized we had cheered the Cub players from different vantage points along the parade route, joining five million people on November 4, 2016.

Tim was on a roll. He told me that he and his brother sat in the stands at the Cubs' first game under the lights at Wrigley Field on August 8, 1988 (8-8-88!). Evidently, broadcasters wore tuxedos to add to the festivities, all except Harry Caray who refused. The Chicago Symphony performed the national anthem on the field. I didn't know any of this.

In the bottom of the first inning, Ryne Sandberg hit a two-run homer, giving the Cubs the lead, but sadly, heavy rain halted the game for a while. Sheets of rain soaked the players and fans alike in the fourth inning; the game was postponed to the next night. I marveled at his recall.

Whether Tim was again at Wrigley the following night during the first full game under the lights (a Cubs' 6-4 win over the New York Mets), I never knew. I figured that somehow Tim had managed to snag tickets both nights.

I called Tim in early October, eager to tell him about my football weekend in Minneapolis. My cousin, Pete, and I had attended a Minnesota Gophers game on a Saturday in late September followed by a Minnesota Vikings game the next day. We sat in the nosebleed section, just a few rows from the top of the new U.S. Bank Stadium. I started regaling Tim with details of the Vikings' 30-17 dominance over the Seahawks, including Kirk Cousins' sweet touchdown passes to Adam Thielen and Justin Jefferson, but he interrupted me. He already knew the Vikings had beaten Seattle. He didn't care about my Vikings.

Tim was far more interested in talking about his beloved Chicago Bears. He was angry about the Bears' terrible loss to the Cleveland Browns, 26-6, the previous Sunday, giving them a 1-2 record. He went on and on describing missed blocks, errant throws, miscommunication between the quarterback and his receivers.

"Who is that Bears QB?" he asked.

"Andy Dalton, I think."

"Yeah, Dalton!" He nearly spat the name.

I worried a little. The more agitated he got, the more difficult he was to understand. Tim took the Bears' losses personally – as if they were intentionally torturing only him.

"I may give up watching the Bears," Tim announced. "They're just awful." Even over the phone, he seemed to be sulking. We abbreviated our conversation.

***

A couple days later, he telephoned me again.

"Hi Tom. I wanted to tell you I just read something great in *Astronomy*."

"What did you read?"

"Oh," he hesitated. "I guess I forgot. That happens sometimes."

"Is *Astronomy* a book?" I wondered.

"No. It's a magazine. I have a subscription. I have one to *Golf Digest* too, and some baseball magazines. Serena helps me order them."

Tim seemed to be trying to pack as much information into his brain as he could before he declined further.

"I'm glad to hear you read a lot, Tim," I said.

"I have lots of time to read, Tom," he explained. "In the morning, it takes me forever to dress, but after I do, I fetch the *Wall Street Journal* outside my door." He was determined to stay current with business news. I wondered whether he followed the stock market, but I didn't ask him.

"I'm reading a lot of travel magazines too," Tim said. "I really hope Serena, Liam, and I will still be able to travel. I'd love to take them to California where I used to live."

"When did you live in California, Tim?" I asked.

"After graduating from Purdue, I got my master's degree at USC, and I stayed with my friend, Scott Dickson. He was a fraternity brother at Purdue. Scott just visited me a few days ago. He had a lot of stories. I had forgotten some of them."

"Scott told me about going to outdoor concerts at the Greek Theater where we sat in the trees – or climbed a tree for a better view," Tim started. "We also saw the Ramones concerts at the Hollywood Palladium. I reminded Scott about the 'mosh pit' near the stage where we pushed other crazy fans around in circles near the stage. That was wild!" "I think we went out at least four nights a week in LA," Tim said.

If Tim had a wild-and-crazy time of life, this may have been it.

"Scott teased me, how I loved going to the beach to watch the Pacific waves and especially the girls in bikinis."

"We went to Vegas too! I couldn't believe all those casinos, all those lights."

"Did you gamble?" I asked.

"Yeah, we played a little blackjack, but I never had much money."

"We went to Sedona too, then drove to the Grand Canyon. Liam would love to see that! Scott wanted to show me all around. We even went to Tijuana in Mexico. Coronas only cost fifty cents there. We had to sleep in a parking lot near a beach somewhere."

"Why didn't you stay in a hotel?" I asked.

"We didn't have much money that night, I guess. I don't think we had a reservation."

"We were always broke," Tim said, "but Scott reminded me that we figured out a way to eat cheaply. Back in LA, we went to a small Mexican restaurant near our place. It had a lot of food during happy hour. So, we looked for empty tables where customers had left half-empty glasses of beer. We sat in their chairs, then headed to the buffet to stuff ourselves. That was just the best!"

I loved hearing Tim laugh. He spent plenty of time thinking about his glioblastoma, coping with his day-to-day limitations, regretting not being able to take Serena and Liam places, worrying about their future, dreading the time ahead when he would get even worse. Scott's visit was the perfect medicine for him.

***

Tim continued to teach me. I was learning about the power of laughter. And with this reflection of his time with Scott, I realized how much Tim's friendships helped as he faced his illness.

I recognize that some people prefer facing a serious disease privately, and I respect that. But I know that I too will need my circle of family and friends to boost my spirits, to share moments of laughter.

9

In early November, I called Serena to schedule my next visit with Tim. She told me that Tim's siblings, Phil and Betty, had visited him. This was the first time all three had been together in two months.

Phil and their dad had marveled at Tim's positive outlook during frequent visits since August. But this time, Tim's mood had changed. He expressed disappointment in people, seemed paranoid, and complained about insignificant matters, saying things he probably didn't intend. Serena was sorry Tim had been in a grumpy mood.

***

When I visited Tim again in mid-November, he greeted me, then introduced me to Liam. Father and son exhibited similar smiles. Liam was quiet as we climbed the stairs. Tim didn't need assistance, but his steps were careful. Sammie followed us into the living room.

I asked Liam about his school, Samuel Osman Magnet School.

"I can walk to school; it's a short walk from our home," Liam said. "Kids in my school are in pre-kindergarten through eighth grade." He told me about his interest in band, basketball, and some of his classes. Liam's politeness and intelligence impressed me.

After enjoying an after-school snack, Liam went to his bedroom to do whatever 10-year-olds do. Tim and I could hear music playing upstairs.

"Did I tell you, Tom, that I've always loved numbers?" Tim asked.

"What do you mean, Tim?"

"I just like noticing curious numbers, such as my birthdate, 11-66."

"Interesting."

"Sometimes I glance at the clock on the wall, and I'm amazed – it's 3:33! Or later I look at the time again, and it's 4:56!!" Tim was excited to share this with me. I'd never known anyone who had a similar fascination with numbers.

I noticed one of the bookshelves nearby and asked Tim whether he had read any good books lately. He told me that he really enjoyed the Babe Ruth book called "Big Fella." Also, Liam had been reading aloud to him, "How You Played the Game," about the life of Grantland Rice, a sportswriter in the early 1900s. He smiled when recalling that Rice was born on an interesting date, 11-11-1880. The book was written by one of Tim's college professors, Bill Harper.

I asked Tim where he had worked after leaving the AMA. He labored in remembering the names of places he had worked, but he knew that many of his jobs were in the healthcare arena. He mentioned being out of work for a while, and also working for a construction company. He shifted his sitting position and nervously moved some papers on the table in front of him. Talking about his work history made him uncomfortable; I moved the conversation to another topic.

I described driving recently through the beautiful highlands east of Pittsburgh to Chambersburg, Pennsylvania, to visit my sister Joan. I mentioned her interests in music and art, her teaching career, and her new home in a senior retirement community operated by the Mennonites.

"Is she your only sibling, Tom?" he asked.

"No, I have another sister, Sue. She and her husband, Dave, live in Rice Lake, in northern Wisconsin. Lakes are beautiful there."

"What's the difference in your ages?" he asked.

Something seemed to be on his mind.

"I'm the youngest. Sue is three years older than I am, and Joan is seven years older," I said.

"Seven years! That's the same as my sister, Betty, and me!" he blurted. "I hardly remember her while growing up," he told me. "I was only 11 when Betty went to college and then she got married."

Tim mentioned that Betty had visited recently. They laughed together, reminiscing. He was delighted to hear Betty's stories about the day he was born, when he caught poison ivy, how he spent hours playing with his GI Joes, and when he was given red cowboy boots, insisting that his mom wash the bottom of the boots every night.

One night when Tim was a kid, Betty recalled getting angry when she was caring for him. She sent him to his room. Not long after that, Betty spotted Tim through the front window, sitting on his bike, carefree and guiltless. He had crawled out of his bedroom window. Tim smiled, hearing that story.

"Were you close with your sisters, Tom?" he wanted to know.

"Yes, pretty close," I replied, "but I think we became closer when my dad died. We had to care for our mom because none of us lived near her. We had to make arrangements to sell the house and find a place for Mom to live."

Tim nodded, thinking about that. "My mom died a few years ago. I wasn't ready for that. We didn't have any warning. She had an aneurysm." He had difficulty saying that word, so he tried to spell it: G-A-R-G-R. Finally, I guessed what he was trying to say.

"Mom's death was really hard on my dad. It was hard on all of us," he said.

"Losing any parent is tough, Tim," I replied.

"My dad is in a care center now, but he visits me sometimes. I bet it's hard for my dad to see me like this."

"Yes, I'm sure he feels awful that his youngest son has been hit with such a terrible disease."

"It's hard not being active, Tom," he said. "I'm used to working, exercising, playing golf, taking Liam to the tennis court, travelling with Serena and Liam, taking Sammie on walks." Sammie lifted his head when he heard his name. We both smiled at Sammie.

"Sometimes, I just can't believe I have cancer. Somedays I feel pretty good."

"Does Liam know about your cancer, Tim?" I asked.

"Yes, Serena told him – but he doesn't know I have glioblastoma."

"Does he talk with you about it?"

"No, not really, but maybe he asks Serena," he said.

"He's really smart, so I bet he has done some research. He helps me all the time, getting things for me, making me feel more comfortable on the sofa, talking with me, reading to me. I couldn't ask for a better son."

"Do you think he realizes that you are dying?" I asked tentatively, hoping not to pry.

Tim was quiet for a long time before answering. "I'm not sure – but Liam is very smart."

Tim shifted gears, telling me that he was trying to exercise. He demonstrated stretches and techniques to strengthen his legs and improve his balance.

When Tim heard Serena come home, his eyes brightened. Serena had returned to work several days earlier. She had timed her Family and Medical Leave Assistance long enough to care for Tim through his radiation. Caring for his needs and driving him to appointments had been a full-time job for months.

"Are you having a nice visit?" Serena asked, smiling.

"Yes, and I've finally met Liam!" I replied. "What a nice guy." I heard Liam come downstairs, eager to greet his mom.

I asked Serena about returning to work after four months.

"It feels good to be back with my colleagues. They have been so supportive since Tim got sick," she said, "but of course, I miss being at home with Tim."

Serena explained that she makes lunch for him each day before leaving, something that he can fetch from the refrigerator or poke into the microwave.

"We're watching Tim's nutrition and trying to limit his snacks," she said, looking over at Tim. He smiled at her.

"How about Sammie?" I asked.

"A wonderful gal, Jessica, stops by to take him out. That really helps."

Tim mentioned that when Serena returned to her job, he watched more television, especially sports. Now and then, he'd find a movie to watch.

Serena added, "We have different tastes in movies. Tim prefers war movies like 'Dunkirk' and James Bond thrillers. I prefer romantic comedies or Netflix series like 'Ozark.'" Tim nodded.

Knowing that Serena was probably ready to fix dinner, I said goodbye. Tim walked with me downstairs to let me out, thanking me for coming to visit.

"I love our talks, Tom," he said smiling.

"I do too, Tim. We'll talk again soon."

I typically turn on the radio while I'm driving, but not this time. My head spun thinking about Tim and Serena, but mostly about Liam.

Liam should be hitting a baseball to his dad in this beautiful autumn weather. He and his dad should be taking Sammie to a dog park. He should be riding the roller coasters at Great America on a Saturday with his parents.

I thought about Tim and his family. They must often be lost in their thoughts, wishing they could enjoy themselves. Instead, they feel isolated. They are coping, but in their own ways, they are already grieving.

10

After returning from visiting Jane's brother and his wife for Thanksgiving in Tennessee, I received a call from Serena, telling me that Tim had been hospitalized. On Tuesday, November 23, Tim complained that he couldn't breathe.

"Something isn't right!" he yelled to Serena, "I'm so uncomfortable."

A chest CT in the ER showed he had bilateral blood clots in his lungs. He remained at Illinois Masonic until November 24, but thankfully, he was home for Thanksgiving.

Several days later, I telephoned Tim. He described panicking when he went to the ER, not knowing what was wrong. Pain medication had helped, but then, he stopped. For some reason, he didn't want to talk about the hospitalization anymore. He changed the subject abruptly – to television news. Sometimes, his mind seemed to jump around; I had to listen carefully.

"Are you watching all this stuff about Trump, Tom?" He didn't give me time to respond.

"I'm so tired hearing all about Trump, the attack on the Capitol, refusing to accept the election results," Tim said, his voice rising with greater intensity. "Did you know, Tom, that he didn't even have the courtesy to attend President Biden's inauguration?"

I changed the subject, hoping that Tim might calm down, and soon after, we said goodbye.

***

Because we were booked with holiday activities, I knew my time to visit Tim would be limited, but we kept in touch by phone during December.

On one call, Tim told me Serena had arranged with his physician to buy a device for his head. He couldn't remember what it was called, but he knew that his head would have to be shaved. Tim dreaded that day. Of course, he knew that many cancer patients lost their hair, so if the apparatus would somehow help him – maybe slow the brain cancer, maybe make him feel better – he was all in.

"When will you get the device?" I inquired.

"I'm not sure, but I think later this month."

I asked him how he was feeling.

"I get tired a lot," he said, "and I've lost a lot of strength especially in my legs. I just can't go on long walks with Serena and Liam anymore. Sammie always walks with them." His speech was still an issue. I had to listen carefully whenever we spoke by phone.

Exercise had always been important to Tim. From the time he played baseball as a kid, he had been in good shape.

"I didn't care about my physique. I just loved being active," Tim said. "Playing outfield, I tried to run after every ball hit my way. In basketball practice, I ran as fast as I could during wind sprints."

"Now this. I mostly sit on the sofa reading and watching TV. When I stand up, I get dizzy. Sometimes, I hang onto things."

"I'm sorry, Tim," I replied. "I'm sorry you're going through this."

"I know, Tom – but I'm doing okay. Really, I'm so lucky. I don't have any pain. Serena and Liam take care of me. Sammie too. We all love each other.
Don't worry about me."

***

During the holidays, I missed being with him in person. Tim had become my teacher. By example, he was guiding me gently, preparing me for the day when I begin to decline. He was teaching me how to cope, to remain optimistic – to face death bravely whenever that time comes.

In all of our conversations, I never heard Tim whine about his diagnosis. I wondered whether I would be as stoic. He was teaching me that confronting his gradual decline with hope for tomorrow and love for others gave him purpose.

11

New Year's Day 2022 arrived. The Hartwell family's celebration was low key, but Serena's sister, Laura, joined them, and December 31 was her birthday. Cause for a party!

I landed two moderating jobs in January, conducted simultaneously over two weeks, on aesthetic enhancements and diabetes. Juggling topics was tough. I breathed a sigh of relief when the final in-depth interview concluded.

***

Driving into Chicago on February 7, I realized how eager I was to see Tim. It had been so long. Ours was an unexpected friendship; we both valued the bond we had formed during the past seven months.

After I rang the doorbell, I waited. This time, Tim was slower to answer. When the door opened, I saw him smiling broadly. He wore the new apparatus on his shaved head – an Optune. It looked like a portable device, a soft helmet with wires connecting it to a battery pack.

Sammie led the way upstairs. Tim paused to rest a little at the top of the stairs. When he sat, Tim talked about the Optune.

"It's really heavy, Tom, but it keeps my head warm. I like that," Tim volunteered. "Serena has to adjust it once or twice per week by moving it slightly on my head."

"Do you wear it at night, Tim?"

"No, not usually. At least I don't think so. Maybe I do. I'll have to ask Serena." Tim's confusion was apparent.

"Do you know how it will help you?"

"It's supposed to destroy cancer cells or slow them from growing, I think," he said. (When I returned home that night, I checked. Tim was correct. It works by creating electric fields that slow down or stop glioblastoma cancer cell division.)

Tim stooped a little to rub Sammie's head. "Aside from my brother and dad, I don't have many visitors, but Sammie keeps me company. He's a good boy." Sammie moved slightly on the floor, nuzzling closer to Tim.

Tim abruptly changed subjects. First, he told me about visits with Phil and his dad, a call from Betty, and hearing from several friends.

Then, Tim told me about his special girlfriend in high school, but that ended when he went to Purdue. Without fanfare, he casually mentioned having been engaged to a woman with two kids. I recalled Tim calling years earlier to tell me about his engagement, but even then, he wasn't sure it would last. Evidently, it hadn't. Serena was the love of his life, and now, she was his attentive, loyal caregiver.

I asked Tim how he and Serena had met. He told me about meeting Serena when they worked at the University of Illinois Chicago in January 2006. He casually asked Serena if she wanted to see a Cubs game; she wasn't sure whether it was a date or not, but she agreed. Wednesday, May 31, they were in the stands together. Magic must have been in the air that day – Tim couldn't even recall who had won. Afterward, they enjoyed conversation at a nearby diner. Two years later, they were married on August 30, 2008. I remembered their wedding vividly.

***

We spent an hour, perhaps two, catching up. He told me about his baseball card collection of several thousand cards. His neighbor, Sam, was helping him with it. As much as Tim was fascinated by numbers, he had special difficulty when citing numbers, so I wasn't sure whether his estimate was accurate or not.

He described dressing up with Serena and Liam for Halloween months earlier, then celebrating New Year's together with Serena's sister, Laura. He loved having Liam home for vacation. Every time he spoke about his wife and son, love radiated through his words and face.

Then, Tim surprised me, asking a few questions. He wondered whether I had been an athlete in high school. I told him I tried basketball and track when I was a freshman, but playing drums in our school band better matched my skill set.

He asked where I had met my wife. I explained that I was a year ahead of Jane in college, Gustavus Adolphus College in St. Peter, Minnesota. When I discovered that Jane grew up in Red Wing, Minnesota, located on Highway 61, I figured this was a good omen. The same highway ran through my hometown, Grand Marais. Tim smiled at that.

I told Tim that Jane and I were members of the Gustavus Choir, even travelling together on the choir's first international tour to Scandinavia in 1967. I explained that Jane is Danish and I'm half Norwegian, so Sweden was a logical site for us to have a serious talk about marriage.

He was curious to know when our children were born, so I told him both had been adopted. Rick had been born in South Korea and joined our family through Holt Adoption Agency when he was just over two years old. He arrived at O'Hare Airport in 1973, accompanied by a nurse. We were thrilled! Friends praised us for adopting a child in need, but we always felt that we were the lucky ones. Tim nodded. He understood.

Then I told Tim that six years later, without warning, Jane received a call from Lutheran Social Services informing her we could meet our infant daughter the *following afternoon* at their office in Eau Claire, Wisconsin. Since we hadn't had any notice to prepare for the arrival of a baby, Jane hustled six-year-old Ricky to the grocery store, instructing him to fill the shopping cart with whatever he thought his baby sister would need while she pushed the cart. Baby food, diapers, stuffed animals, toys were tossed into the cart. Ricky thought of everything for his baby sister, Jamie!

Tim grinned. He seemed to be imagining the joy Jane and I felt when our children arrived. Over the months, we had focused so much time talking about Tim's life, his family, his interests. I viewed Tim's interest in my life positively.

I promised to see him again soon. I did, three weeks later.

12

On February 28, something changed that affected the remaining time Tim and I had together. After sitting in my usual chair, I spoke first:

"Tim, I know you still read a lot. Are you able to write?"

Tim smiled broadly. "I write like I talk – not so well! Why do you ask?" His eyes twinkled.

I had been pondering this during my hour's drive to his home that morning. I kept thinking of Tim's family, but especially about 11-year-old Liam. Our grandson, Grant, is the same age. He and Liam are both smart, sensitive, and inquisitive. I couldn't imagine Grant coping with the terminal illness and eventual death of his dad, Rick.

"Well, Tim," I started. "We have been having incredible conversations for six months, since you became ill last August. Don't you agree?" Tim nodded.

"How about if I take notes as we talk, then when I get home, use those notes to write letters from you to Liam?"

I waited for a reaction. Nothing. I wondered whether Tim understood what I had said, what I was proposing. Still nothing. Perhaps he hated the idea. Finally, he replied.

"Do you mean to give Liam when I'm gone?" he asked softly.

"Yes, Tim. If you wish."

He didn't hesitate a second. "Oh, Tom, that would be great! I love the idea!"

We decided to keep this as a surprise from Liam and Serena. I could tell, Tim relished the intrigue of sharing the secret.

And so, I pulled out a lined notepad, ready to take notes as we talked. I maintained eye contact with Tim as best I could as he spoke. Now and then, I asked Tim to repeat something. When he had difficulty saying a word, he tried to spell it, but that didn't work well either. I concentrated on understanding what he was saying, while capturing his feelings, his emotions.

When our visit ended, he and Sammie again walked with me down the stairs. I reminded Tim to keep our secret! His smile was broad. Then he surprised me, "I love you, Tom."

***

When I arrived home, I immediately sat at my desk ready to draft Tim's first letter to his son. Oh yikes, my penmanship had seen better days! *Guess I need to look down at my writing every now and then.* I proofread, printed, and saved a copy in my Word file – "Hartwell letter 1."

February 28, 2022

Dear Liam,

My friend, Tom Toftey, is going to help me write some letters to you. I hope you will like reading them. I wish I could write them myself, but Tom will help me.

Today after school, you're playing basketball at your school. Mom is going to watch you play. I wish I could be there, but I will hear the score when you get home.

You are 11 years old and in the fifth grade. You started at the school when you were very young, maybe preschool. You love it there, and I am so proud that you get "A's" all the time.

Someday, you'll go to high school – maybe Walter Payton H.S. I would love that! Maybe someday you will play basketball in high school. Doctors say you might be 6'6"! Wow! I only grew to be 5'9".

I always hoped you would play baseball and maybe you will someday. You will have my most valuable baseball cards. Right now, you don't show much interest, but in time, you will understand the value.

My Lou Gehrig card is my most valuable card. I also have a Mickey Mantle card that I bought for $15 when I was a teenager. I would like to get a Babe Ruth card, even if it is in bad shape. I have Ted Williams, Willie Mays, Yogi Berra, Roger Maris – so many! Our neighbor, Sam, is helping me with my collection; I trust him.

You may want to keep my best cards – or you may want to sell them.

Oh – Sammie just came upstairs. He is the best dog in the world!

Love,
Dad

Looking at the rest of my notes, I decided to confine each letter to one page, so that when they were placed in a three-ring binder, no letters would be back-to-back.

Depending upon how long I visited with Tim on a given day (often determined by Tim's energy), I realized that some visits may result in a few letters, while longer visits may result in many more.

I was determined to capture Tim's exact language, when possible, while interpreting his intent as well as I could. This would be a challenge.

Satisfied with the first letter from father to son, I started a new letter.

February 28, 2022

Dear Liam,
I think about what sports you might do in high school – maybe baseball and basketball, but maybe tennis. Since you are left-handed and will be tall, tennis would be a great sport. But Liam, I want you to do whatever you like, whatever makes you happy!
I played saxophone in school. You play the trombone, and you have a friend who plays trombone too. Sammie likes the sound. I love the fact that you enjoy playing trombone.
And – you sing all the time! Maybe you will sing in a group in high school.

Sometimes, I wonder where you will go to college. And I wonder what you will study in college. You like cold weather, so you may go someplace local or nearby. You have so many interests – and you are much smarter than I am. You can do anything.

When I was in college at Purdue, my first year was bad. Sometimes, I skipped classes. I fell behind, couldn't catch up. I should have studied more. I tried a sport – baseball – 85 people tried out, and I made it through the first day with 15 others, but then I didn't make the team. I was a little disappointed. I could hit the ball. I think I played as well as the others. But it is hard to play Division I sports. Then I realized: "You are a college student now!" I started studying.

After graduating from Purdue, I went right to USC – the University of Southern California – for my master's degree. It's a lot of work. I worked and worked! I always remember watching USC sports on TV. I really like USC and the warmth of Southern California.

Love,
Dad

Focusing on academics, sports, music, being involved, staying active. These were common themes in Tim's hopes for his son.

In my bones, I shared an ache of regret with Tim, not knowing where Liam would go to high school or college, what he would study, what profession he would choose. He hoped his words would someday help Liam weigh his options, always remembering *"You can do anything."*

I imagined Liam reading these letters for the first time, feeling the warmth of his dad's dreams for his son, the depth of his love. Liam would be comforted, but he would miss his dad.

I again looked at my notepad – still more notes! As I reviewed my penmanship, I could hear Jane speaking to me, *"When you write fast, it's illegible."*

Then I reread my remaining notes. They were not meant for Liam; they were meant for Serena. Without permission from Tim, I decided that Tim should leave letters to Serena as well. I had no doubt that he would agree.

February 28, 2022

Dear Serena,

My letters to you – thanks to my friend, Tom – will be the result of my talking with him in person or by telephone. I told him that I am lucky he comes to visit me, because not too many others visit.

I awoke this morning, maybe 5 a.m. – feeling so good. No pain in my head. I am so lucky.

I showed Tom some of the woodworking my dad did. I look at his woodworking, thinking he could have been an engineer. That wooden tower with the steel balls is so creative. (Tom tried it out.) He is 92. His vision doesn't work well now.

Serena, I want you to know that you are just the best wife. You help me so much.

I'm glad that we will be joining Fourth Presbyterian Church in Chicago next month. This is better than using my old church in Prosper. And – I am so pleased that you and Liam will be baptized.

Love,
Tim

The affection and gratitude that Tim had for Serena continued in every conversation I had with Tim.

When Tim told me that his wife and son had agreed to be baptized, his face radiated a joy that I seldom saw during my visits.

Growing up, Tim and his family had been active in Grace Lutheran Church in Prosper.

Serena mentioned that her family didn't regularly attend a church. Her dad may have occasionally attended a Methodist church. Her mother was Pentecostal, always wearing dresses, never being allowed to dance. Serena viewed these strict edicts as "oppressive."

Tim started attending St. Paul's UCC on Fullerton Avenue, but Serena didn't feel a sense of community there. He wanted all of them to worship at the same church, so they continued to search.

Finally, at Fourth Presbyterian Church on Michigan Avenue, they found a church where they felt welcome. Even worshipping on Zoom, people made the Hartwell family feel included. When Tim said this church "is better than using my old church in Prosper," he may have envisioned his funeral or memorial service in Fourth Presbyterian. He may have imagined Serena and Liam, his dad and siblings sitting in the front pew.

Writing these first three letters from Tim gave me a peaceful sensation that I was helping his son and wife cope with their deep, eventual loss. I hoped I was reflecting the depth of Tim's love and hopes for Serena and Liam.

I told Jane about the secret Tim and I now shared, and she smiled, understanding the importance of my visits with Tim.

13

March 10, 2022. I stopped at a neighborhood Dunkin' Donuts before beginning my drive into Chicago. Donuts are my weakness, especially sugar raised.

"Not nearly as good as the World's Best Donuts in Grand Marais," I thought to myself as I took the first bite. A writer for the *New York Times* travel section had written about the donut shop some years ago. He concluded, "The donuts in Grand Marais claim to be the world's best – and they just might be."

I hoped that Tim would feel well today. Instead of feeding him a question from my list, I decided to see what was on his mind as I continued to take notes. I vowed to write larger, more legibly. That would pay dividends when I translated his words into letters.

Tim answered the door with Sammie by his side. We didn't even reach the top step when Tim blurted, "Tom, do you remember our secret? I may have slipped!"

"That's okay," I replied. "Maybe Serena didn't hear you or understand what you were talking about. Maybe she will forget what you said. It will be a long time before Serena sees all of these letters." Tim nodded, hoping so.

As I sat, I explained, "Tim, I have written three letters from our last conversation, two for Liam and one for Serena. I decided that some of your letters should be to Serena because of what you say. I hope that's okay with you."

"Yes, that makes sense."

"Before we begin talking today, I want to read each letter aloud. While I read this first letter to Liam, please interrupt me if I've made a mistake, and I will correct it. If everything is okay, I want you to sign it in your handwriting."

I read the first letter. Tim listened carefully. He understood this letter was from him to his son. He concentrated as I read. At times, he smiled.

"Oh Tom, this is wonderful. I don't have any corrections," Tim said. After pausing, he continued, "Someday, Liam will read this letter. Maybe he will read it aloud. Maybe he will read it quietly while lying on his bed late at night. Maybe he will read it over and over. I wonder how long it will be before he reads it."

Tim's eyes looked past me, thinking, imagining. I remained quiet.

"Okay. Are you going to read the next letter, Tom?" he asked.

"Yes, in a minute, but first you need to sign this letter. Here, I'll help you." I placed the letter on a hard surface in front of him, handing him a pen.

"Where do I sign?"

"Right here, under the word 'Love.'"

"What do I say?"

"You don't need to say anything, just write 'Dad.'"

"Dad?"

"Yes. This letter is to Liam, and you are his dad, so you write 'Dad.'"

"Where do I write that?"

"Right here where my finger is – under 'Love.'"

"Dad?"

"Yes."

Others have said that Tim was meticulous, that he feared making mistakes, that he became anxious when faced with a difficult task. I was witnessing this. Tim looked up at me then down at the letter, gripped the pen tighter, and wrote "Dad." He looked back at me smiling.

"Was that right?"

"Yes, Tim. It was perfect."

I read the next letter aloud to Tim slowly. When I read about Liam singing all of the time, Tim smiled broadly, interrupting me.

"He does! He sings all of the time. I can hear him singing upstairs when he's in his room." Tears formed in his eyes.

"I'm already thinking about how much I will miss Liam when I am gone, Tom."

I nodded. I couldn't speak. As I age, my emotions rise to the surface more frequently than they used to. After pausing, I read the rest of the letter. Again, Tim didn't have any corrections, so I placed the letter in front of him to sign.

"Where do I write my name?"

"Here. Under the word 'Love.'"

"Tim?"

"No, write 'Dad'" because this letter is also to your son, Liam.

"Oh yeah."

In order to help Tim, I wrote "Dad" and "Tim" on a scratch paper, then covered up "Tim" pointing to "Dad."

"That helps," he says. *Why hadn't I thought of this earlier?*

He signed the next letter to Liam carefully spelling D-a-d.

I assured him that he signed just fine. Then, I began reading his letter to Serena while Tim listened carefully, interrupting me only once as I read.

He smiled, "Yes. I said that! My dad is one of the smartest people I know. He could have been an engineer or a doctor or anything. He is so smart, Tom."

"If you don't have any corrections, Tim, you can sign this letter to Serena."

"Where do I sign?"

"Under this word – 'Love'."

"Dad?"

"No. This time just sign your name – 'Tim,' because Serena is your wife," I answered, pointing to my scratch paper.

"Just Tim?"

"Yes."

"Under 'love'?"

"Yes – perfect."

A half-hour had lapsed, but Tim seemed able to continue. He slowly walked to the kitchen to get a glass of water. When he returned, I showed him a black three-ring binder I had bought.

"I'll keep all of the letters in this binder, Tim." He approved, smiling.

"This will be a great surprise for Serena and Liam," he said. "I can imagine them opening the binder for the first time, wondering what this is – then starting to read the letters. I bet they will smile a lot, maybe even laugh. I hope so."

Tim was anxious to create another letter. I didn't guide him with another question. He had something on his mind.

March 10, 2022

Dear Serena,

Thank God, I married you, Serena!

I remember that time we had in Lake Geneva when I played three rounds of golf by myself. I was playing really well, but then suddenly, I shanked my ball to the right over and over. I knew something was wrong.

I recall talking to the guy in the golf shop – wondering whether I could just hit some more golf balls. I told him that I had started to hit my ball poorly, and I knew something was wrong with my speech. He probably thought I was drunk or just acting stupid, but he let me hit some more balls.

Then, I remembered driving you and Liam.

[He stopped to correct me, "You should say "on that Friday" so I added that.]

Then, I remembered driving you and Liam <u>on that Friday</u>. I wanted to buy something to celebrate how well I played. I knew something was wrong with my speech.

Back at the hotel, my head really hurt. I started crying – I knew something was really wrong. This was the first time I had cried since my mom died.

You couldn't understand me. You called my friend, Shaun. I think you got me to the hospital in Lake Geneva, but it was small and not able to help me much. Shaun talked with you. He kept you together. Shaun suggested that you get an ambulance to take me back to Illinois – maybe Lutheran General Hospital. Shaun's friend did my surgery.

(In December) you got me the thing for my head – the Optune. You shave my head and then move the thing on my head as you are supposed to do. This will add time to my life. Granted, I didn't like to have my head shaved, but it's working. My head never hurts! I wake in the morning, and my head doesn't hurt! You help me so much.

I don't know how many months I have, but I'm praying that nothing is growing. Of course, I know that could change tomorrow.

Just know that I love you, Serena!
Tim

Tim's memory of Lake Geneva was vivid. Undoubtedly, he had told the story many times to friends. Some details were fuzzy, but he covered the trauma of that Friday well.

As he said "I don't know how many months I have," he spoke matter-of-factly. He remained realistic, even stoic.

Tim took a sip of water, shifting slightly on the couch to become more comfortable. Sammie stirred beside him on the floor, sensing Tim move. Tim looked at Sammie lovingly. My pen was ready. I wondered where our conversation would move as I took notes.

March 10, 2022

Dear Liam,

> *Sometimes you and Mom and I take trips. We always take Sammie. He goes with us everywhere. We never leave him.*
>
> *My memory isn't so good on all the places where we've gone. I should ask your mom all the places where we've been.*
>
> *I think we went to Michigan once – maybe Traverse City. I couldn't believe how beautiful the water was. Maybe I played golf, but I'm not sure. The golf isn't as expensive as it is in Illinois.*

I remember driving to Iowa. I really remember that trip. It's not far from Chicago. We went to that Field of Dreams ballpark (in Dyersville). That ballpark is really great!

Oh, I remember running the bases with you and Sammie. We ran and ran around those bases. That was really something! The day was in the 60s. We had so much fun. Everything is free there – parking, seeing the ballfield, running the bases.

I'd like to go again to the Field of Dreams. Maybe if your mom agrees, instead of being buried in cement, my ashes could be scattered on the Field of Dreams someday.

Love,
Dad

He spoke so casually, so calmly, "…instead of being buried in cement…"

I wondered whether he and Serena had talked about this. Did she know about his wishes? Had she thought of where Tim's ashes should be buried? Should I tell her? I decided against it. This was too personal. I was confident Tim and Serena would discuss this.

Tim was ready to resume our conversation.

"Oh, I know what I need to talk about next, Tom," he said. "Last night was just the best! We did something all together."

I was pleased to see how easily Tim adapted to the adventure of creating letters for his son and wife. We had formed a partnership, but this was Tim's surprise.

March 10, 2022

Dear Liam,

I went to your band concert last night. Mom was so glad that I made it. The concert was upstairs four levels and there was no elevator. It was really hard work for me to walk that far – but I made it! Mom was angry that there wasn't an elevator for people like me.

The music was great! You play the trombone really well. I loved the band concert.
Even Sammie likes to hear you practice playing your trombone.

But – I might be ready for a nap today.
You know how much I love golf. You tried golf a little, but you haven't had lessons. Golf is expensive, but if you decide to play golf, lessons will be important if you want to get good at it.

Love,
Dad

Tim was proud that Serena was upset the school didn't have any elevators. "Isn't that against the law?" he mumbled to himself. But Tim didn't dwell on that. All he knew was that he had made it, climbing up four floors – and he had done it without help! He smiled jubilantly.

I envisioned Tim slowly climbing to the fourth floor, finding the effort and determination it took. This had been an incredible challenge, and he had conquered it!

Without warning, he fired a question at me.

"How old are you, Tom?"

"I'm 76, Tim."

"Oh, I didn't know you were that old!"

"Good to know," I replied, smiling.

"That means – let's see…you're how much older than I am…?"

"Twenty-two years older."

"Oh, wow. You're a lot older."

That thought had crossed my mind many times. Tim was young – 54 – and I was so much older, but as months of conversing flew by, our age difference didn't matter. We felt like we'd been good friends for a long time. Ours was an unexpected friendship that neither of us anticipated when we sat together in the AMA cafeteria, plotting our next sports prediction.

Our age difference was the reason we didn't socialize together after working at the AMA. I was anxious to take the train home, to see Jane and our Shih Tzu, Digger. Tim was single.

We walked together down the stairs, following Sammie. Tim and I said goodbye, and he again thanked me for writing the letters. Sammie came over for a final scratch around his ears. I leaned down, and Sammie gave me a little lick.

"Isn't Sammie just the best, Tom?"

"He sure is."

"I hope I didn't spoil our surprise for Serena."

"Don't worry about it, Tim. It's okay if you did. Someday, Liam and Serena will love reading your letters."

Tim nodded as he closed the door, probably still worrying that he had flubbed the surprise.

I was eager to tell Jane about my conversation with Tim, the range of topics he covered, and his excitement in working on the letter project. She was my confidante. A month or two passed before I told anyone else about the adventure Tim and I had undertaken.

14

Nearly two weeks had lapsed since I had seen Tim. Jane and I had driven to Michigan to celebrate our granddaughter's golden birthday in mid-March.

On March 23, Serena met me at the door. She was heading into work a little late. I was happy to see her. She appeared preoccupied, but I imagined her days were hectic – working, caring for Tim, spending time with Liam, taking Sammie for walks, doing various chores around the house. She told me that she had a camera in the living room, so she could check on Tim from work anytime, and she confessed to taking a frequent peek.

Although my black binder was under my arm, Serena didn't seem to notice. Worry was on her face that morning as she left for work. *Was it worry because of changes she was seeing in Tim? Was it worry for Liam as he listened to his dad speak? Was it worry from something at work?*

Tim greeted me with a smile, obviously pleased to see me again. I read aloud the three letters from my previous visit, and Tim signed each carefully, following my instructions. He did NOT want to make a mistake. I showed him the black binder which contained his first three letters, now paper-punched. He smiled proudly. As I grabbed my notepad, ready to write, Tim began talking. He had been looking through a travel magazine that morning, and saw photos of places in Los Angeles where he and his friend Scott had visited: Hollywood Boulevard, the glitzy stores of Rodeo Drive, homes of movie stars, the Pacific Ocean beach.

As he paged through the magazine, he talked about other places he would like to visit.

"My family didn't travel very far when I was a kid," he said. "My dad didn't get a lot of vacation time, so we went to campgrounds, but we always had fun." Tim continued to page through the magazine.

"Just look at all of the national parks, the deserts and mountains and cities…" His voice trailed off.

Sometimes, Tim's eyes looked past me as if I wasn't really there. I learned to avoid interrupting his moments of solitude.

March 23, 2022

Dear Serena,
 I look at the map of the United States sometimes, wishing I could go places.
 I'd like to go to Seattle or Portland. They have some of the best baseball fields.
 I've never been to Stanford University. I like everything about California. I've seen the Redwoods once. They look fake – but oh, my gosh! I hope you and Liam will see the Redwood trees someday. Maybe we could fly out West then rent a car. We could drive to Tucson and Phoenix.
 Also, I wish we could take a drive to the East Coast. That would be so much fun.

Love,
Tim

Tim paused, evidently thinking about something important.

"You know, Tom, we're not going to be able to travel like that, because Sammie always goes with us, and he could never ride on a plane. But I like to think about things like this."

I felt sad for Tim, knowing that he wouldn't be able to explore more of our beautiful country with Serena and Liam. Tim had so many hopes for his future with them, but he continued to be realistic as the months passed.

March 23, 2022

Dear Serena,

Last night I almost cried. I looked online for a baseball player who was able to play with brain cancer, and I only found one guy who had it. And he may have already died.

If I had to guess, I think I will live for another year, maybe a year and a half. I'm feeling great. I'm eating well. I'm exercising.

Serena, you are so smart. You are keeping me alive.

I don't fear dying, especially since I am more tied in with a church again.

Dying is out of my hands. Everyone dies eventually.

But I worry about you, Serena. Maybe when I die, it will be easier for you. You do so much for me. You and Liam are as close to each other as you can be. This will be wonderful after I die.

By the time Liam is done with high school, you will be able to retire. You might retire then or work a little longer. You'll figure out what to do.

Love,
Tim

I later researched baseball players who had glioblastoma. Between 2003 and 2022, a flurry of Philadelphia Phillies died of glioblastoma, sparking an investigation of Veterans Stadium. Radar guns and the field's surface were under suspicion. One who died, in 2004, was Tug McGraw (father of country singer Tim McGraw) who ranked among the best relief pitchers playing for the New York Mets and the Phillies.

In my research, I couldn't find a major league player who had been able to play with brain cancer, only a long list of those who had died from the disease. When I researched others who had confronted glioblastoma – entertainers, authors, artists, and other athletes – the list was sobering. Life expectancy seemed to be 12-16 months, but tumor genetics appeared to offer some variability.

Nearly every time we visited, Tim mentioned that he didn't know how long he would live, but he usually threw out possibilities – including the hope of living several years.

Tim's Christian faith was strong, surfacing especially when talking about his family. I didn't see Tim cry very much, but when he did, it wasn't because he was dying. He was crying at the thought of missing Serena and Liam, of not being a part of their future. At those moments, I shared his deep regret, his profound sadness. We sat in silence, wiping our tears.

***

I wondered – how will I someday face my last months, my death? If I am hit by a serious illness, I too will have day after day, hour after hour, thinking of Jane, already missing her deeply, worrying that she will be okay, but knowing that our children will care for her.

I will think of Rick and Shelley, Jamie and Patrick, wishing I could follow their activities and careers. I will regret not being a part of their lives while they enjoy their challenges at work, their retirement years, hearing about the joy of watching their children and grandchildren thrive, their travels to foreign lands and discoveries in this country, sharing laughter and memories.

I will miss watching our five grandchildren grow and flourish. Grace, Megan, Grant, Declan, and Hazel – what an amazing array of beautiful, talented, intelligent, and loving grandchildren. I will regret not being able to share in their special occasions – their musical and sporting events, graduations and college visits. I will miss weddings, career decisions, the births of babies or perhaps, a decision to adopt a child.

As a Christian, I am promised eternal life. I know this. But as comforting as that is, I will miss earthly relationships. My wife, our children and their spouses, our grandchildren, our relatives and friends.

March 23, 2022

Dear Liam,

I think about your future sometimes. Maybe after high school you will go to Northwestern University. That's a great school, and you're smart enough to get in. You are so close to your mom, and Northwestern would be close to her.

You're so good with your hands. Maybe you will go into civil engineering.

Architecture would be cool. You are so smart – much smarter than I am.

I hope you won't be a lawyer. I hate lawyers!

You are sharing my medical experience with me. Maybe you will admire doctors. Perhaps you will go into medicine. Or you could be a professor at a college or university.

You can do anything, Liam.

Love,
Dad

Tim had thought about possible careers for Liam to consider. I winced a little when Tim said that he hated lawyers – no idea what prompted that – but that was Tim. He spoke his mind.

Before leaving, I showed him the black binder again, pointing to the clear pockets inside the front and back covers.

"Tim, don't you think you should put something in these pockets? What would Serena and Liam like?"

Without hesitation, "Photos! Photos of our family from our trips. Of our families and friends! Maybe a photo when Serena and I were married, or photos of our parents. Oh, a photo when Liam was a baby and little guy! We'd better include a photo of Sammie – maybe one of him when he was young. And we'd better have a photo of all of us together. How many photos can we have, Tom?"

"I don't know, but we'll figure it out, Tim."

"Maybe a photo with my mom, dad, Betty, Phil, and me. I don't know if we have one with our dog." Tim was genuinely excited about this twist to the surprise he was planning.

Great idea," I replied. "Where can I find some photos that Serena won't miss?"

He looked around the room, then his shoulders sagged and his face tightened. He thought for a long time, then frowned, "Oh, I don't know. I forgot. I have no idea where Serena keeps the photos." Disappointment overwhelmed him. I thought he might cry in defeat.

Thinking quickly, I said, "How about another idea, Tim? I could buy some cards for various occasions, you could sign them, and then on the outside you could write whether each card was for Serena or Liam, and you could write when it should be opened."

Tim was quiet, still dejected that he didn't know where to find photos.

"So, Serena and Liam will open these cards after I'm gone?"

"Sure," I said, "One card could be for Serena's next birthday, another for Liam's. Another card for your next wedding anniversary. Maybe a card to Serena and Liam for Christmas. Maybe a silly card just for Liam to open anytime. How does that sound?"

"Good idea, Tom. I like that! I'll find some money so you can buy the cards," he said, pausing. "Oh, I don't know where Serena keeps money."

"That's okay, Tim, don't worry."

Satisfaction was visible on his face. He had forgotten about the photos. He thought about leaving special cards for Serena and Liam.

We had enjoyed our time together, but it was time for me to start my drive to Winfield, and I was leaving Tim in a positive mood. As always, Tim was gracious in thanking me for visiting him. He and Sammie ushered me down the stairs to their entry way.

Seven months had lapsed since Tim's cancer appeared. I knew he counted the months, remembering Dr. Muro's prediction that he would likely live for 12 to 14 months. I counted them too.

15

I was eager to visit Tim again, but Jane and I were busy with Holy Week activities at our church, St. Paul Lutheran in Wheaton. We had been members since 1983. I enjoyed singing in the church choir for Maundy Thursday and Easter services.

On April 21, I waited longer for Tim to get down the stairs to open the door, but when he did, I felt welcomed by the customary Hartwell smile. I quickly realized his speech had declined even further. I didn't know what he said, but I pretended. He seemed to labor more climbing the stairs, stopping once midway. His face seemed puffier. He had gained weight, perhaps due to medication.

When we began visiting, I told him how surprised I was to notice he had entered the Masters golf pool. He grinned. I suspected he may have done that for my benefit, to see whether I would notice. We compared notes on the golf tournament, whining a bit, then laughing. Neither of us had fared very well in the pool. Out of 19 entries, I had finished in 13th; Tim finished even lower.

After reviewing the letters from my previous visit, he was anxious to begin talking.

April 21, 2022

Dear Liam,

You probably know that I grew up in Prosper, a couple hours west of Chicago.

My dad worked hard and so did my mother. Dad only had two weeks for vacation each year, so we didn't go on too many trips, but when we did, we took our camper to a campground somewhere.

My brother, Phil, and I would throw a baseball around and if there was a lake nearby, we'd go swimming. Phil and I really liked our vacations with our mom and dad.

A highlight for our trips was finding a restaurant where we could get something to eat.

My mom was a good cook and talented seamstress. She could write really well. When I was in high school, she worked outside the home. I think she worked in an office.

I remember that my mom had stomach issues at various times. She was born in the early 1930s and died at age 86. Her funeral was at Grace Lutheran Church in Prosper where we had attended.

My dad was a hard worker in his job. He was so smart. He was a talented wood worker. Now, he is 92 years old. I don't get to see him very much.

My parents were good parents. They taught me a lot.

Love,
Dad

Whenever Tim shared memories of his family with me, he spoke with affection. Theirs was a close, loving family. He admired his parents' work ethic, their skills, their obvious love for their children.

The kids were typical siblings. Phil teased his younger brother, and they both teased their older sister. Betty remembered sitting between her brothers in the back seat as they drove to a campground. Phil and Tim taunted Betty, taking off their socks, playing with their feet which they named "Stinky" and "Smelly."

Betty was disgusted at their antics, but also laughed at her younger brothers.

April 21, 2022

Dear Liam,
My brother and I had a lot of fun growing up.
From the time I was 6 or 7, I played baseball. (I bet you're not surprised to hear that!) I played in Little League, mostly in the outfield. Phil played on the same team – third base, I think.

When I was 15, I used to join my friends swimming near Prosper. We'd walk about an hour to get to the swimming hole. I could swim okay. As least, I didn't drown!

When I was young, I read a lot – mostly about sports. Some books I would read in a day or two. I don't think I ever read mysteries.

Of course, I also played baseball on the Prosper High School team – mostly center field. We had a 50-50 record, I think. We only had one really good pitcher. I considered playing baseball at Purdue, and tried out for the team, but I didn't make it. I was really disappointed.

Love,
Dad

Tim's eyes smiled whenever he described his childhood years. Back then, folks didn't always lock their doors. He and his pals hopped on their bikes to head everywhere – to the swimming hole, baseball diamond, or playground.

One of their favorite places was a wooded area behind his home with a large gully, perfect for hanging a garden hose from a tree, then swinging over the gully. Tim smiled, thinking of those carefree days.

16

I learned from Serena that her dad, Chuck, had come to care for Liam during his school's spring break. Serena appreciated his help while she worked. Serena's mom remained in Florida, because she was terrified of testing positive for COVID. According to Serena, her dad wore two hats: Mr. Mom, taking Liam to band practice and fixing dinner, and Project Manager, tackling small projects around the house."

Chuck was amazed Tim didn't seem to be fazed by the disease. More than once, he told Chuck, "I feel good. How could I have a brain tumor?" When Chuck shared Tim's comment with Serena, she spoke directly to Tim: "Believe me, Tim, you really do have a brain tumor."

***

Tim and Sammie greeted me on April 25. Tim seemed upbeat, eager to visit. As we climbed the stairs, Tim mentioned that Sammie had been sticking close to him. Wherever he was, Sammie was with him.

I read the letters from my previous visit to Tim, and he approved. Signing his name continued to be an effort, but he never complained. He wanted to sign each one.

Then, I displayed the greeting cards I had bought for Serena and Liam to open on special occasions. I had several options, so that Tim could select his favorite birthday cards, a special anniversary card, a Christmas card, and one that Liam could open on any occasion. I had asked a young clerk at my nearby CVS if I could see some valentines that the store had in storage since February had long passed, but he didn't know where to look.

Tim took his time selecting each card. He was careful in signing, asking for assistance in knowing where and how to sign his name. Then he wrote a different message on each envelope: "To Liam – to open on your next birthday." "To Serena – to open on our next wedding anniversary." He sealed each envelope. Tim was determined to complete this task perfectly.

Looking pleased, he placed each envelope in the binder's see-through plastic pockets. He felt Sammie rub against his leg, perhaps regretting that he didn't have a card for Sammie.

Why hadn't I thought of buying a card for his pal, Sammie?

"I think Serena and Liam will like these cards," Tim said. "The funny card you found for Liam is great. I bet they will be surprised. I wonder whether they will keep them. I bet they will."

"I bet they will too, Tim," I said. "They will probably look at them every time they read through the letters from you."

April 25, 2022

Dear Liam,

When I was a kid, I had a dog – I think her name was Tiffany. She was mixed breed and half size. You would have liked her. She was a good dog.

She ate inside. One day, when we were on vacation, she was tied up outside and a kid let Tiffany loose. She was hit by a car! All of us cried and cried while my dad drove. That is the worst thing in the world for a kid, when a pet dies.

Sammie is about 8 years old. My dad found him somewhere. Since I've been sick, someone takes Sammie for a walk every day. When I lie on the couch to take naps, Sammie comes upstairs and lies down on the floor next to me. He never jumps up on the couch.

Sammie is the best dog in the world, don't you think, Liam?

Love,
Dad

Losing our dog Digger was tough. Pets join a family. A lovable bond is formed.

Serena told me Tim's dad found two-year old Sammie in a Tennessee shelter when he was full grown. In 2017, the Hartwells met Sammie for the first time, and a year later, he was theirs. Liam was just seven years old. It was love at first sight for Liam and Sammie.

April 25, 2022

Dear Liam,

My sister, Betty, lives out East – where they talk funny! She isn't able to see my dad or me a lot because of the distance.

As you know, my dad is 92 and lives in a nursing home. My dad calls me sometimes; more often, I call him.

When I was at Purdue, I remember that I went to Disney in Florida with my folks. At night, my dad snored like a bear! We had fun going on rides at Disney. Phil didn't go on this trip; I think he was married by then.

I really love my folks.

Love,
Dad

Tim thought about his parents, his siblings, his childhood and high school friends. He thought about his best friends, Drew and Scott. They called him on the phone, but he missed seeing them.

Tim spent hours alone in his thoughts, sometimes all day, until Liam came home from school and Serena finished work. Without human interaction, he was lonely.

April 25, 2022

Dear Liam,

I like astronomy. One of my goals is to use our telescope to see Saturn some night.

I should have used a telescope when I was in high school. I think I may have enjoyed astronomy as a job, but a PhD would have been important, and I don't think astronomers make too much money.

My dad never looked at the telescope. I don't think Phil looked at it too much either, but when he did, he probably used it to look at people instead of the stars.

Someday, maybe you and your mom may enjoy it – looking up into the heavens.

Love,
Dad

One evening at 3 a.m., Serena and Liam heard Tim noisily lugging his dad's old telescope onto the roof deck. Looking at Saturn was on his mind! Although they managed to get it upstairs, they had difficulty setting it up. It was just too complicated. Serena vowed to buy a new one.

April 25, 2022

Dear Liam,

The Cubs had a great game the other day, winning 21-0 – but then Pittsburgh won three out of four games. Suzuki looks great though.

The White Sox are in trouble. I loved the Dodgers when I lived in Los Angeles while attending USC.

I can't watch the Bears anymore; I like college football best. USC could win the national championship this year with their new coach.

Love,
Dad

Tim loved listening to Liam report the day's sports news, especially about his Chicago Cubs. He wanted to remain current. He loved spending time with his son.

This was what I remembered about meeting Tim at the AMA. He could talk about sports for hours, I was convinced. I imagine that he was a fine athlete, but he was also a loyal fan. He loved to attend sporting events, and his passion was evident as he watched sports on TV

April 25, 2022

Dear Serena,

> *We are joining the church on May 12, I think. We were supposed to join earlier, but then Liam got COVID.*
> *We watched church on TV for Easter.*
> *People are nice at the church. You have a friend from work who goes there. We can park nearby for only about eight dollars – and we can leave the car there for hours.*
> *I tried six or seven different churches, but they didn't seem right. Some only had a few people attending. Who pays for that?*
> *I need to walk to build up my strength, but I must be careful about the stairs.*
> *The other day, we took a long walk. We took Sammie with us and walked for an hour and then later, we walked for seven-tenths of a mile in the same day. That was a very good day.*

Love,
Dad --- Oops! Tim

Tim was horrified that he had made that mistake in signing the letter to Serena, but when I suggested that he just cross out "Dad" and write "Oops," he laughed aloud. He was in good spirits.

Exercising was so important to him. Knowing that he and his family enjoyed taking two lengthy walks made him feel strong and healthy.

April 25, 2022

Dear Serena,

I don't know if I have six months to live, a year, a year-and-a-half, or three years. I see the doctor every few weeks.

May 4 will be an important day when I see the doctor. She will look to see if my head works. Is the tumor growing? Is it shrinking? Is it gone?

I am so lucky. I wake up with no pain. I'm in a great position. I'm tired a lot but not in pain, but the last two days, my stomach has been killing me. The chemo pill makes me tired. And when I go to bed, I fall asleep easily.

Serena, you couldn't be any better! Oh, my gosh, Serena, you work so hard – taking care of me and Liam, your job, everything at home. You do everything! You don't want me to do too much because I get dizzy when I stand up.

I think about how hard it would be if we had more than one child – but I am so glad you will have Liam to love and care for. You and Liam have such a close relationship – oh, my gosh! Liam loves you so much.

Since I have no pain, I am hoping the tumor will be gone when I see the doctor.

I love you,
Tim

Tim and Serena faced every medical appointment with hope, anxiety – and yes, dread. As much as they wanted to be optimistic, they suspected that Tim's brain cancer had not improved. Tim hoped that his tumor had not grown. Without any head pain, he would be happy to live a long time like this. May 4 was circled on their calendar.

Tim was reflective for a few moments. Before leaving, I sensed he had something important to say in another letter.

April 25, 2022

Dear Serena and Liam,
I have no fears about dying. My friend Shaun says that the pain won't be bad at the end – and then it will be gone.

What are my hopes for you when I am gone?
This is hard to think about.
I hope you will both be safe, happy and joyful!

Love,
Tim & Dad

17

Knowing how important Tim's appointment on May 4 had been, I called him the next day. Tim was home alone as usual, but we didn't talk too long. He seemed tired. Not really down. Just fatigued.

Tim was anxious for school to be over, so that Liam could be with him during the day while Serena was working. Just hearing Liam practice his trombone upstairs or sing with his radio made Tim feel better.

May 5, 2022

Dear Liam,

You'll be done with school by the end of May or maybe early in June – just one month to go! I am so proud of you. You have perfect grades. You could have skipped a year of school, but your mom and I thought this could mess you up socially and emotionally.

You know that I love the Cubs, but they are so bad right now. They just lost two straight games to the White Sox.

I had my doctor's appointment yesterday. She spent forty minutes with me and your mom and says that I "am a little worse." She said it's hard to tell, so I will see her again in three weeks. I'm not sure whether I'll be getting new meds or not. She said the side effects can be scary.

My balance has been a little better lately. I feel fine sitting, but weak when I'm walking. I need to do something to strengthen and stretch my legs, so that I can walk with you, Mom and Sammie.

Love,
Dad

After Tim's appointment, Serena texted me that Tim was beginning palliative care. I wasn't sure how that differed from hospice care, so I did a little research.

Palliative care can begin while treatments are still being given, but hospice care isn't typically started until after treatment of the disease is stopped.

A part of Tim's palliative care was initiating treatment of M-VASI, used to treat brain tumors that are resistant to previous treatments. It was administered as an infusion into a vein every two weeks.

An assortment of side effects is associated with M-VASI, but Tim's only side effect was extreme fatigue.

Tim was talked-out but asked me to stay just a little longer. Perhaps he didn't want to be alone. He wondered whether Jane and I had traveled internationally.

"We've been very fortunate, Tim," I said. "I think we may have visited 25 countries."

"Wow! That is great," he said, smiling. "What was your favorite?"

"Ah, that's tough," I replied. "We loved all the Scandinavian countries and the majestic Alps of Switzerland and Austria, but we were in awe seeing the Pompeii ruins in Italy. We also spent several memorable weeks in Korea where our son was born, and we visited St. Petersburg, Russia, with my men's barbershop chorus."

Tim was quiet for a brief time.

"I hope someday, Serena and Liam will be able to take an international trip," Tim said. "I wonder where they will go." His eyes looked past me, somewhere far away.

I hated to leave Tim. His loneliness was visible.

18

I thought about my previous visits with Tim. He had been unusually talkative. I had drafted more letters based on our conversations during my last few visits than at any time. Sometimes, I felt as if Tim stored information in his brain prior to my arrival that he wanted to share in his letters to Serena and Liam. As months slipped by, this continued.

May 9, 2022

Dear Serena,

I think about my last doctor's appointment. She (the doctor) doesn't know much about my tumor growth. I guess we'll learn more at my next appointment in three weeks.
If I get a pain in my head, it will be hard to read, so I'm trying to read a lot now.
During the last few days, I've been getting up at 5 a.m. I read the newspaper, make coffee, feed Sammie, watch CNN on TV for an hour or so. Sometimes, I watch a movie. It takes me a long time to get dressed, maybe 40 minutes.

Sometimes I take a nap when I'm feeling really tired.

I love you, Serena!
Tim

After the letter's closing, Tim wanted to sign this letter, so that it would read, "I love you, Serena!" I thought that was sweet.

I'm unsure whether Tim had always been an early riser. Perhaps his medications caused him to awaken so early. Having an early-morning routine was important to him, and I suspect that routine gave Serena some comfort.

May 9, 2022

Dear Liam,
I'm halfway through a book about Scott Carpenter who was one of the astronauts. Being an astronaut would have been awesome. My friend at USC wanted to be an astronaut, but you need a lot of science classes to be considered. Maybe 1 out of 20,000 make it.
I had the perfect height (5'9") to be an astronaut – but not the right brain!

Before deciding to go to Purdue, I thought of Michigan State University because they had great basketball teams. I also thought about Iowa and the University of Illinois, but I think I only visited Purdue. You love cold weather, so I bet you won't go to college in California. Maybe you'll go nearby, like Northwestern. Or maybe the U. of Illinois. I hate the University of Michigan – but I admit, it's a good school.

When I was in high school, I had a girlfriend. When we went to college, we broke up – just too far from each other.

Tom looked through my yearbooks from Prosper High School. If you look at them someday, you will find a photo of us in my senior yearbook. We went to a "turn-about dance" together and had our picture taken. I look so young.

She was so nice, but it wouldn't have worked out. It hurt me when we broke up, but it was good that we did. I probably wouldn't have gone to USC if we had stayed together. Thinking back, we should have broken up before we did.

Love,
Dad

Tim's interest in astronomy certainly led to his dreams of being an astronaut. In addition to Scott Carpenter, Tim mentioned reading about other astronauts during our conversations. He admired their pioneer spirit, their sense of adventure, and the impressive preparation necessary in becoming an astronaut.

May 9, 2022

Dear Liam,

Of all the seasons, when I was your age, I loved summer the best. This was when my friends and I went swimming, played baseball, went boating. I don't think I ever tried waterskiing though.

I'm trying to remember, Liam – did we ever go to the Great America amusement park? Maybe one time. I hope we did.

I remember going to friends' birthday parties. Sometimes, we'd stay overnight at each other's houses. Lots of laughing and joking late into the night!

During those times when our family went camping, we'd find a good campsite for our camper. One of my favorite things was roasting marshmallows over the fire – burned were the best. Then, we'd add Hershey candy bars and put them in Graham crackers to make s'mores. They were SO good! Roasting hot dogs over the campfire was also fun.

I remember going swimming one time that was scary. I don't know where we swam, but there was a current that kept pushing me out further into the lake. I was swimming alone – which isn't smart! I hoped that someone would see me. I didn't learn how to get out of a current by swimming sideways along the shore. When I finally came home, I was breathing so hard. I could have drowned. I still think about that time.

Love,
Dad

Isn't it interesting what vivid childhood memories we have? Sitting around a campfire, burning marshmallows, salivating for a s'more. Oftentimes, it's the little things that spark a memory!

When I recall my childhood, I think about picnicking with my family on "The Point," a picturesque jut of land near the Coast Guard Station and lighthouse in Grand Marais. It's a magical place even now. I loved sitting on the flat rocks, just watching the waves of Lake Superior, feeling their rhythm. I learned when the glaciers melted, the landscape was at the surface again. The Point is one of the only places on Earth where a person can stand on surface rock which is 1.1 billion years old.

After Jane's primary students returned from a winter skiing vacation in Aspen or a spring trip to Florida, she asked what they had enjoyed most. Even though they had likely seen many sights, experienced many adventures with their families, they often replied, "Swimming in the hotel pool." It's the little things we remember.

The terror of nearly drowning haunted Tim. He retold this story several times during our conversations. I wondered whether this may have occurred while living in Los Angeles and swimming in the Pacific Ocean, but Scott Dickson doubted it. Tim would have shared his fear of drowning with Scott. Perhaps this happened while swimming in Lake Michigan where rip tide currents are common.

May 9, 2022

Dear Liam,

You know that I played a lot of baseball. When I was in high school, I also went out for football and basketball.

I shouldn't have tried football. I wasn't that big. I hurt both of my shoulders. I also broke my foot and wrist. It was stupid for me to play football.

Until my senior year, I played basketball. Then, I decided to focus on baseball. I was too small for basketball, and we had a terrible team. I think we only won three or four games.

I got an award in basketball, maybe because I had ONE great game. But we had a super player who should have gotten the award. He was three times the player I was.
My friend, Sam, keeps trying to sell less valuable baseball cards from my collection. I have Mickey Mantle and Lou Gehrig for you to have. My goal is for him to find a Babe Ruth card in good condition. The company he uses,
PNS, sucks. Sam is getting angry at them. So am I.

Love,
Dad

I left that day overwhelmed, thinking what Tim will miss by not being a part of experiences with his son and wife – not sitting beside Liam at a Cubs game or cheering him on at a tennis match or basketball game, not joining a standing ovation after his band concerts, not taking Serena on a surprise silver anniversary trip, or celebrating their golden anniversary at a gala party with family and friends.

Perhaps I was experiencing survivor's guilt.

19

May 16, 2022

Dear Serena,

I remember when we met. We were working near each other in similar work. You helped me get work from other companies related to cardiology. You really helped me. Even though I was dating someone, as I got to know you, I really liked you.

Our first date was to a Cubs game. I bet you could tell that I liked you a lot. You were cute, trusting, believing, and very smart. I don't even remember who won the game! I think you were dating someone at the time, but he was a bad person. He treated you very poorly. About a week later, you called to tell me that you were done with him.

We went on other dates, but I can't remember where we went. I wish I could remember. But I recall that we went to the Indy 500 with friends. We may have had a lot to drink.

When I asked you to marry me, I didn't get down on one knee – and you were disappointed. But you said, "Yes!" I felt so happy. We talked about a wedding date sometime in the future.

Our wedding was beautiful. You looked so wonderful when I saw you for the first time, when your dad walked you down the aisle. He was funny! He gave me a hug and a laugh. We had such a great time. You were so pretty in your wedding gown which was beautiful. I felt bad that I didn't have a chance to talk to some people who left early, and I remember being upset with one of my cousins who was angry about something.

We went back to the place where we were married to have dinner. That really brought back memories. You sent the restaurant a nice gift for treating us so nice.

Our honeymoon was amazing! We went to Hawaii – staying at the Hilton Hawaiian Village in Honolulu on Oahu, but also to Kauai and the Big Island. We also stayed with a friend from my days at Purdue to save some money. I think we were gone for three weeks. I think I played a little golf during our honeymoon. Hawaii's golf courses are the best. You were probably hanging out, enjoying the beach. We were so happy to be in Hawaii.

I love you so much,
Tim

As Tim and I were visiting, Serena overheard our conversation. She recalled sitting in the stands at Wrigley Field on that first date, cheering on the Cubs.

I asked Serena where Tim had proposed.

"On the top of the Hotel Washington in Washington, D.C.," Serena answered. "He was nervous."

Smiling at Tim, she added, "We went to Hawaii on our honeymoon, and about ten years ago, he took me back to Kauai and Oahu. This time, Liam came too. He was just one and a half."

"Tim, I heard that another friend visited you recently," I said. "Who was it?"

"Dave Farlee stopped over," Tim answered. "We worked together years ago, but I forgot where."

Serena was still listening. "You and Dave worked at the American Academy of Pediatrics in the mid-1990s," she called from the kitchen.

"Oh yeah."

"What did you talk about?" I asked.

"Dave reminded me that he and my friend from grade school, Drew, had taken Liam out to shoot some hoops one day while I was napping. Dave, Drew, Scott Dickson, and I had all been close friends for years, going to baseball spring training in Arizona, playing golf, and heading to the Indy 500! Dave thought we went to Indianapolis about 20 times."

Tim smiled as he recalled their early trips to Indianapolis, arriving in time to enjoy Saturdays drinking beers around a campfire. In later years, they arrived as early as Thursday in order to get a spot in Lot Two across from the racetrack, away from the rowdy people.

I was amazed, not only about Tim's recall of details, but also how easily I could understand him. His ability to speak clearly seemed to vacillate. Perhaps I had become a better listener.

"Dave really made me laugh when he told me about the time when we unpacked our stuff. He and Drew and Scott always gave me grief about how picky I was when I packed my gear for the trip." Tim began laughing, telegraphing a memory.

"Once, after arriving, when I set up my folding chair, they howled when they realized I had brought Liam's folding chair instead of mine." "About how old was Liam then?" I asked.

"Probably three years old." Tim chuckled at the memory.

May 24, 2022

Dear Serena,

I really wish we could go on a trip – a vacation to the West Coast or the East Coast, some place we haven't gone before. We've never left Sammie though, and that would be hard.

We'd fly and then rent a car. You would be scared for my health. You wouldn't want to be far from a hospital, I know.

We went on a vacation to northern Wisconsin once. It was gorgeous – the sky, the water – so cool. I wonder whether we ever got to see the northern lights.

I talked to my brother yesterday. I told him how scary my illness is. I'm alone with Sammie. He must think this is easy.

With your job and me, you are too busy to drive me to see my dad. And on weekends, you need to relax. I understand that. Oh my gosh, Serena, I am so lucky to have you and Liam. You are keeping me alive.

When I die, it won't hurt – not like how my head used to hurt. The pain will be gone. I keep praying that my talking and walking will be fine. I pray every morning, thankful that I don't have any pain.

You are the best – I love you,
Tim

As Tim's health declined, frustration and anger surfaced occasionally. Serena told me that his friends noticed this, even while speaking with him on the phone.

His agitation fluctuated in late spring and seemed to increase as summer began.

Tim told me he and his brother had been close as kids. "We kind of drifted apart in high school when we had different circles of friends," Tim said.

"Then, we were off to college and the beginning of our careers."

Was this Tim or was this his disease distorting his thinking?

Tim told me that his brother is a teacher, and I remembered what that was like. I shared my recollections with Tim while he listened intently.

"Teaching was my first career," I said. "I taught for eleven years, but it isn't easy."

"What happened?"

"I burned out. I taught English and journalism, so my students wrote a lot of papers, and there's no time during the school day to evaluate them. Jane and I had two young children then, and I realized I was hurrying through dinner because I had so much to do." Tim listened intently.

"Maybe Phil will burn out, but maybe he won't. How did you decide to stop teaching?"

"I loved teaching, but I knew something had to change. So, I conducted an experiment: I assigned an essay for my junior English students and a feature story assignment for my journalism students – each about 2-3 pages long. I wanted to see how long I spent reading each assignment a couple of times, noting errors in grammar, spelling and punctuation, suggesting changes, then writing a comment at the end of the paper, assigning a grade, and recording it in my grade book. I figured that evaluating each paper took an average of 13 minutes. And that was times 130 students."

"That's a lot of time, Tom. I never thought about that when I went to school. I wonder if Phil has that much work," Tim said.

"Very likely, Tim, but teaching every subject and grade level is different," I said. "I've had four careers. Teaching was the most difficult – but also, the most fulfilling." Tim thought about that. *Teaching was the most difficult – but the most gratifying.*

I continued, "When I left teaching, my next job was in public relations. I worried that I would miss teaching terribly, that I had made a mistake. My new boss also had been a teacher, and he told me when he entered the business world, he realized that there are a lot of teaching moments in various types of jobs. He was right."

***

Before I left, Tim had something else on his mind. He tore a page from my tablet, then asked for my help. He wanted to write a special note for Serena – something that she could keep and reread.

He wanted to be sure his spelling was correct.

The note was lovingly simple:

I love you!

20

June signaled an important change for Tim: Liam's summer vacation began, so Liam would spend more time with him. Even if Liam was busy online or reading books, he was nearby. Tim felt comfort in knowing Liam was with him.

I wonder whether males view human interaction differently than females.

According to Serena, Tim and his dad could sit in the same room together for an hour, without saying a word – and be completely content having spent time together.

My dad was editor of a weekly newspaper. When I was a young teen, I worked at my dad's print shop on Saturdays sweeping the floors, dusting the display cases, and restocking shelves while my dad did job printing: letterhead, envelopes, posters. Printers' ink was everywhere; the shop was always a mess. During the fall, we listened to the Minnesota Gopher football games on the radio. We never said much during our time together, but I always felt very close to my dad during those Saturdays.

My good friend, Jerry, recalled attending a party with his wife, Merrie. When they returned home, Merrie chastised him, saying, "Jerry, your friend so-and-so was at the party, across the room from you, and you never said a word to him!" Jerry replied, "Yes, I did. He nodded and I nodded back. That was enough."

June 2, 2022

Dear Liam,
    I remember the day you were born. How beautiful you were! You were already tall – maybe 10 feet tall! [Tom: Yes, that's what your dad said!]

I was in the hospital when you were born. I remember worrying about your mother. This was such an exciting time – but scary too! I'm not sure I slept very well when you got out of the hospital after a day or two. I remember that you were crying while we drove home. But when we got you home, I couldn't have been higher with joy!

I recall that I got in trouble for holding or moving you incorrectly.

I was out of work for about a year then, but when I started a new job, it was tough for me to walk Sammie. I should have taken more time off to help your mom with everything, but I was so worried about my new job. I know your mom did 90% of the work with you – and she didn't like it that I wasn't helping more.

Now – you're growing taller. You're not taller than I am yet, but your features (like your feet) show that you will be very tall. You're already smart, and I bet you will be smarter than Mom and me.

You'll have a great summer vacation – maybe playing more tennis, maybe even trying some golf!

I know you worry about me, but I just hope you have a fun vacation.

I love you, Liam!
Dad

I could have kicked myself! When Tim told me that Liam was ten feet tall at birth, I laughed aloud, and Tim joined me. I should have realized, he meant to say that Liam *weighed* ten pounds (and six ounces) at birth. I wasn't sharp enough to think of that.

I remember calling Tim after Liam was born. He was excited and so proud to be a dad. He had married at age 42; he had become a father at age 44.

June 2, 2022

Dear Liam,

Some old photos of my dad have surfaced from when he was in the Korean war (1950-1953). There are some good ones of him and his buddies. I wonder whether he kept in touch with any of them over the years.

I don't think he told me very much about his time in this war. If he was in conflict, he very likely didn't want to talk about this. For lots of veterans in various wars, it is too emotional to talk about the war. I hope you never have to fight in a war.

Did you know that we talked about having you skip a grade when you were young? You were certainly smart enough, but my friend, Shaun, convinced us that the negatives outweigh the positives.

It's amazing that you have been in your school since you were a three-year-old and will stay there through the eighth grade. Then, it will be off to high school! Maybe at Walter Payton High School which has a great reputation.

Love,
Dad

I wasn't surprised that his dad hadn't shared experiences from his service in the Korean War. I have two close friends who served in the Vietnam War. I'm certain they saw combat, but neither has shared any details from those days. I suspect their memories are still raw.

June 2, 2022

Dear Serena,
I'm really tired today because of the three medical visits I had yesterday. Phil took me for the first time. Maybe this gave him a better idea of what I go through.
Yesterday's appointments involved a lot of stopping and waiting in three different offices. I think the infusion took three hours. All of this is mentally tiring.

I feel fine now – no pain – but I might be gone in 1½ years.

Love,
Tim

Tim became somber.

"I really don't know how much longer I have, Tom," Tim said. "I try to stay positive, but I can tell that I don't have a year or three years left even though I say it. I don't tell Serena and Liam that, but sometimes, things seem different inside me."

"I understand Tim," I said. "I'm so sorry."

We sat quietly for a moment. Then I said, "You are so young compared to me. I have already lived a full life, and you should be looking forward to so many years to spend with Serena and Liam. If I could trade places with you, I would."

That touched Tim. His tears moved slowly down his cheeks. He didn't even wipe them before speaking. "When I die, there will be a service at our church in Chicago. I hope you will come."

"Of course, Tim. Jane and I will be there."

"Will you speak at the service? You have gotten to know me so well, Tom," he said, still emotional.

"I will be honored, Tim." I was touched by his request, and my tears began.

"I love you, Tom."

"I love you too, Tim."

21

When I visited Tim on June 10, he seemed content. He had slept well and had eaten a good breakfast. Liam was busy reading upstairs. Sammie was asleep nearby.

Tim was excited to tell me that Scott Dickson had come from California to visit him for a couple of days. They enjoyed talking about those years when they lived together. He told me about their conversation. They reminisced about their Thanksgiving tradition: buying carnitas burritos, taking them back to their condo, then watching a marathon of "Twilight Zone" episodes during the entire day.

Scott confessed to Tim that when he first learned Tim had brain cancer, he worried how Tim would handle it. He thought that Tim might continue to whine "why me?"

When Tim told Scott, "I'm going to fight this. Don't worry about me," Scott wasn't convinced. Over time, he learned that Tim meant it. Tim felt good hearing this from his friend.

Scott admired how well Serena cared for his friend. He marveled at her stamina and positive outlook, even when he saw that Tim was sometimes demanding.

"You won the lottery when you married, Serena," Scott told Tim.

"I did, Tom. Scott was right," Tim said.

June 10, 2022

Dear Serena

We're going to take a drive to Lake Geneva in a few weeks, just to relax. We're going to have fun.

I'd like to go again to the Indy 500. I think I've gone about 50 times. It is so much fun.

You were going to take me to hit a few golf balls. I can't do it. I can't walk well – my legs feel so weak.

I don't think I'll play golf again. Maybe I could putt the ball at the driving range. I think Liam will go to the driving range sometime, maybe this summer. If he's interested, he should take some lessons. I had golf lessons, and they helped so much.

I'm trying to remember; did you play sports in high school? I think so. Maybe gymnastics.

Love,
Tim

Tim was understandably frustrated by his memory loss. He tried so hard to remember Serena's sports. (I later learned from Serena that she had not been a gymnast; her sports were volleyball, basketball, and track.)

Tim got his wish! On June 16, 2022, Serena, Liam, and Tim returned to Lake Geneva for an overnight stay at The Ridge ten months after their last visit. Of course, Sammie joined them.

Serena removed Tim's Optune for the day, freeing him from the device. They drove to Geneva National where Tim's first indication of brain cancer appeared. They lounged by the hotel pool, enjoying pizza, sitting in the jacuzzi. That night, they listened to a live band in the hotel.

Serena had booked a room with a patio overlooking the lake and pool, so Tim could sit outside, enjoying warmth from the sun and a gentle breeze. Sammie snuggled beside Tim.

This time, they left Lake Geneva on their terms.

***

Increasingly, Serena had difficulty concentrating at work. She was thankful to have the remote camera in the living room, allowing her to check the screen frequently.

With urgency, Tim called Serena whenever he was confused about something. Occasionally, the alarm in the Optune battery made a sound, and that frightened him. Serena explained that either the cable had become detached or the battery needed charging. Tim didn't know what to do. Serena told Tim to just turn off the Optune.

June 10, 2022

Dear Serena and Liam,

Your baptism is coming up soon. I'm so happy you will be baptized. The church (Fourth Presbyterian Church, built in 1912) is so beautiful.

Love from your husband and dad,
Tim & Dad

Knowing that Serena and Liam would soon be baptized gave Tim an inner peace.

June 10, 2022

Dear Serena,

I'm so lucky. I know I nearly died at least three times. I could have died in Lake Geneva on the golf course. I could have died driving the car.

The pain was so bad in the front and back of my head one morning at 4 am, I couldn't breathe. I pleaded to you to take me to the doctor now! The worst pain was in the hospital, and the nurse didn't believe me. I could have died. Finally, finally I got help, and I stayed for two nights.

We haven't talked about when I die. Not yet. You are only 48, and I want you to be happy. If you need to meet another man someday...but...but...I don't want to think about that. We haven't talked about this yet.

I pray sometimes. I don't have pain – and I thank God for that.

Love,
Tim

Tim's greatest fear was pain. Any pain. He often recalled the terrible pain when he had brain surgery, but also the pain experienced in November when he was hospitalized in the middle of the night from pulmonary embolisms. Occasionally, he had stomach pain, but what he feared most was any pain in his head.

As soon as I asked Tim whether he and Serena had talked about Serena's marrying again, I regretted it. I still kick myself thinking about that. He looked back at me with such a strange look when he said, "I don't want to think about it." He may have been thinking, "*I can't think about it.*"

June 10, 2022

Dear Serena
    I call my dad sometimes, but he doesn't talk too much. He might have some friends where he lives. I hope Phil sees him a lot.
    I don't hear from many people from high school. I'm not going to worry about it. I don't think people write letters anymore. Some old friends may not even know about me.

Love,
Tim

Over the months, Serena and Phil reached out to Tim's high school friends, but I sense that when Tim went to Purdue then to USC for several years, he left Prosper behind. On one level, Tim understood that many high school pals may not have heard about his disease, but he still had hope that his friends from 35 years ago would rally around him.

Tim wondered why some friends or colleagues didn't at least send him a card. He guessed that some folks didn't visit because they might feel awkward. He also knew that the fear of testing positive for COVID kept some from mingling with others.

In reading about the effects of brain cancer, I knew that the disease causes memory issues and confusion. I had witnessed this with Tim during my visits. While Tim focused on those friends who hadn't contacted him, I questioned how many calls or cards he received that he didn't mention to me. I wondered who had visited him that he hadn't recalled. We talked honestly about this, and he acknowledged that his brain cancer was causing memory problems. He could have forgotten about some friends who had written or visited him.

Tim and I spent some time discussing the difficulty folks have when visiting someone who is critically ill. What do we say? How do we begin? We may hope the person hospitalized will lead the conversation. In our discomfort, we may hope the visit is brief. We acknowledged that we too had neglected visiting or contacting someone who was ill, who could have valued having a friend visit.

If a relative or friend is facing a terminal illness, we may feel at a loss for words. Our anxiety increases. When saying goodbye, "Feel better soon" or "get well" don't seem right.

Tim and I agreed that simply making the effort to visit, to just be there, to sit next to the loved one, to hold the person's hand is enough. With repeated visits, our comfort level improves.

***

During my teaching days, I conducted a survey among my high school English and journalism students. I asked each student to rank-order the difficulty of 20 communication tasks from very easy to very difficult. Ranking "very easy" was "yelling at my younger brother (or sister)." No surprise there. Ranking "most difficult" was "giving the valedictory address at graduation." The thought of giving a formal address in front of a thousand people was terrifying for them. Ranking somewhere in the middle of the survey was "participating in a small group discussion" and "meeting one of my parents' friends for the first time." Interestingly, ranking second most difficult was "introducing myself to a foreign exchange student."

Because my students were adolescents, I didn't consider including "interacting with someone in the hospital" or "visiting with someone who has a terminal illness" in the list. I wish I had.

22

I called Serena in early July to arrange a date for my next visit. She told me that she was noticing significant changes in Tim. His behavior was taking a drastic turn, becoming unpredictable. Serena described his brain as suddenly short circuiting. He was easily confused and agitated. Occasionally, he acted normal and rational, then he would do or say something that made no sense. She related several examples:

Liam had decided to take the week off from tennis camp, to stay with his dad while his mom worked. Early in the week, while dragging his Optune battery pack across the living room floor, Tim yelled at Liam, correcting him on the steps for turning on the TV and the speakers. Liam was correct, but Tim's loud insistence frightened Liam, so he called his mom at her job. Serena suggested that he go upstairs, lock his bedroom door, and FaceTime with her until she arrived home.

Once, Tim tried to pour milk instead of water into the Keurig reservoir. He used color names to distinguish TV channels such as "2 red 6 channel." While strolling with Serena in the courtyard in their building, he suddenly started walking toward busy Fullerton Avenue.

Serena and Liam became increasingly worried about this sudden change in Tim's behavior. He used his toothbrush on his face as if he was shaving and used pump soap instead of lotion for his skin.

Serena finally removed anything from the bathroom Tim might ingest, thinking it was food. She also removed anything that he could use to harm himself or them.

Although Serena worried that Tim might turn on the oven, he never did.

Serena had always monitored Tim's medicines. Some prescriptions kept him awake, until 2 a.m. or even later. And when he did sleep, he often awoke early.

Serena asked Tim to stay in bed until at least 5 a.m., and he did – spending early morning hours reading or writing. *Yes, writing.*

On one visit, Tim showed me a story he was writing about a fictional road trip. He told me he had researched potential locations for his characters. He wanted me to read the story. I looked at several pages, but his handwriting was difficult to decipher, his sentences incoherent, his spelling so poor that understanding his plot was impossible. I complimented Tim but suggested that I'd rather spend the time visiting with him.

His fascination with numbers increased. He took delight in realizing that he and Serena had been married on 8-8, that Liam was born on 10-10, that his brain surgery had been performed on 9-9, that Sandy Koufax's career with the Dodgers had ended in 1966, the year that he had been born.

July 8, 2022

Dear Liam,

My friend, Tom, stopped by today to visit, and you answered the door. I heard him tell you that you had grown since he last saw you. I believe that!

You told him that you're playing a lot of tennis – I'm so happy. You also mentioned your interest in baseball – maybe even Little League someday. But when Tom asked, you said you weren't so interested in playing golf!

When Tom asked how your grades were, you humbly told him that you didn't think you had gotten any B's. Wow – all A's! I am so proud of you, Liam.

You, your mom, and I plan to take a little trip in August for two or three days to Lake Geneva. I really look forward to that!

I love having you home during the days now that school is out. I try to take a nap each day. If I forget to take a nap, the next day is usually bad.

When Tom was here, you went upstairs for a while, then you showed Tom some books you like – all nonfiction. One huge book was called "Exploration of Nature." Another was "How to Survive Anything." And you also told him that you liked looking up stuff in the Almanac.

I just loved hearing you and Tom talking.

Love,

Because of Tim's increasing discomfort, I no longer asked Tim to sign each letter. I didn't want to increase his stress one iota. He didn't notice.

Although Serena had warned me about Tim's anger and loud outbursts, I never witnessed any of these during my visits.

When Tim mentioned how thrilled he was to listen to the conversation between Liam and me, I was reminded of my mother, who lived to be nearly 105. Occasionally, I sat with her as she joined other residents during mealtime at the care center. I conversed with a couple aides at our table. Mom preferred to listen to our discussion, but later, commented on what we had said. She didn't miss much!

Tim so looked forward to returning to Lake Geneva for another visit, another chance to relive the beauty of that small tourist town next to the lake. He didn't want Serena to drive too far; this trip would take only 90 minutes.

July 8, 2022

Dear Liam,

I'm glad it is summer, so you are home while Mom works. My high school pal came once or twice. He and I went to Purdue University together. I don't hear from other friends from high school. They may not even know I am sick.

I am so lucky I don't have any pain. I remember my surgery long ago – a burning pain, stupid burning for a long time. I had to be awake during surgery to answer questions. I remember that a guy was monitoring me – while I was in pain. He told me that this pain is worse than dying.

My friend, Shaun, was there with your mom. Were you there too? I wish I could remember. But I am glad you're here now, Liam.

Love,

Tim's irritability was heightening. I could hear it in his voice as he spoke. I could sense it in his face; he smiled less frequently. He seemed to be less comfortable sitting on the sofa.

I felt bad that those around him were seeing a different Tim because of his brain cancer. But as soon as he spoke about a regret, a disappointment, Tim spoke of the love around him, the care that his wife and son gave him. He spoke of his dad's visits with his brother, understanding that visiting him was difficult for them. He spoke of getting calls from Drew in Florida and Scott in California.

Sometimes in our conversations, Tim worked to beat the beast of his disease by talking about the joy in his life.

July 8, 2022

Dear Serena,

I just love the house we found to live in. I think we looked at about six houses before buying this one. Our neighborhood is pretty, and our neighbors are nice. We're close to stores too.

I feel good that we don't have to worry about money, even though we make less money now since I am sick.

Your folks are awesome – they are so nice. They really brought you up well. I told Tom that you have a sister who visits a lot.

Even though your family didn't go to church when you grew up, now you and Liam are baptized, and that makes me feel great. At the (private) baptism, I was glad that my dad was there, and also Phil and his wife Rose. The church is so beautiful. People there are so welcoming.

I think we went out to eat after the baptism, but I am not sure. I am so happy that I was there.

Thankfully, I am in no pain, but I'm really tired. I'm trying to avoid making stupid decisions like eating at the wrong time – but sometimes I get that wrong.

I just hope I can keep living. I know it will be harder for you when I die – harder than it will be for me. You and Liam will figure things out.

Love,

Serena confirmed later that Tim's energy started to fade noticeably during the baptism, so his fatigue after the service was understandable. The family dined at the Cheesecake Factory, but Tim remained very quiet.

Was he recalling sitting in a pew witnessing the baptism of his wonderful wife and loving son? Was he smiling at his family as he watched them eating together? Was he already missing those he loved so dearly?

July 8, 2022

Dear Serena,

I am so glad we're going to take a drive in August – maybe to Lake Geneva. I hope the weather will be perfect. I hope we can find the perfect place to eat, sitting where we can look outside. You have found great places to eat before.
You don't like to drive too much, but you do okay. Maybe we can drive around, maybe visit the golf course where I used to play.
I think you may be able to take this thing (the Optune) off my head, since you take it off sometimes. You adjust it every week. It feels so good on my head, nice and warm, but it is a bad design. It is so heavy. How can a small person handle it? But it helps me.

I'm still living – and still living without any pain! I am so lucky.

Love,

Whether or not Tim recalled the family's trip to Lake Geneva in mid-June, I wasn't sure. Looking forward to another trip clearly energized him.

Throughout July, Tim asked Serena several times whether she had canceled the August trip. As much as he looked forward to returning to Lake Geneva, perhaps he suspected that he no longer had the energy to travel.

July 8, 2022

Dear Serena,

My next MRI is coming soon. I am really scared, and you probably are too. I hope my doctor will tell me the tumor hasn't grown – but I worry. I don't know whether I will get better or not, but the appointment will scare the heck out of both of us.

Sometimes, I just get tears thinking about you. You are so smart, so kind, so helpful to me. It's hard for me to expect any more from you! Why have I been able to live so long -- you.

You get depressed sometimes. I try to remind you that we have been lucky to have been together this long. It's hard not to cry, thinking about how quickly I could be gone.

Love,

Tim faced his final MRI with trepidation, and he knew that Serena did too. Serena told me about a memorable day.

Tim's fear was understandable. He was smart enough to understand how much he had declined since that day he shanked the ball at Geneva National. He used to be able to take long walks with his family. He used to be able to stretch and exercise, to push himself. He used to be able to concentrate while reading. Now, fatigue was his companion. And fear was joining his family.

Tim rarely cried, but on July 12, the day of his final visit with the neuro-oncologist, Tim just wept and wept. Serena held him tenderly. Her tears joined his. He knew he was deteriorating each day. He realized he was dying.

He had so much hope, but reality hit him that he was leaving his family. He wept deeply, sorrowfully that day. Serena felt broken. If Liam was nearby, she was unaware. Perhaps Liam was in his room. If so, he may have heard his dad sob, and he may have been aware that his mom was weeping. And he may have cried himself, knowing.

As Serena held Tim, she told him that she and Liam loved him. She assured Tim that they would be okay.

July 12, 2022, was one of the worst days of Serena's life.

She told Tim that it was okay to let go when he was ready.

23

I first heard about the concept of giving a loved one who was nearing death, the "permission to die," in 1991.

My dad's cancer hadn't been caught early. It metastasized, and he declined quickly. When he was rushed to a Duluth hospital 100 miles from home, my mother, sister, and I stayed with him for 11 days. I thought he would die in the hospital three times. We were surprised one morning when Dad's physician told us we could take him home, as long as a hospital bed could be moved to the ground floor of our house. He was giving Dad a gift – being able to spend his final days in his home.

Prior to getting his cancer diagnosis, my dad was invited to be featured in the first one-man art exhibit in a newly opened art gallery in Grand Marais. Of course, he was honored, but he declined, suspecting that he was ill.

Since he was now home, my sister, Joan, said that she could organize Dad's art exhibit using paintings that were in local residents' homes. My mother had meticulous records of who owned his paintings. Working with a local art committee, Joan went to work. Soon after Dad returned home from Duluth, his doctor visited him. As I walked outside with the doctor, he told me that my dad would likely die within three days. I wasn't surprised, since he was so feeble. Still, hearing the words was tough. I told him my dad had been looking forward to seeing his art exhibit, scheduled to open in a week.

When the doctor heard that, he revised his prediction – he would live for a full week following the opening. Accompanied by the county nurse, my family joined Dad in viewing approximately 50 of his watercolors and oil paintings on the afternoon before the exhibit opened. We wheeled his wheelchair around the gallery, stopping so that he could view several paintings at a time. As weak as he was, he reveled in seeing every one of his paintings again.

During that next week, artist friends visited him, telling him which paintings had been their favorites. He heard every word. He smiled as they spoke and replied when he was able.

One visitor was George Morrison, one of America's finest Native American artists. He and Dad spent a lengthy time together. Dad had been George's mentor, encouraging him as a teenager to pursue his talent and passion. In 2022, George Morrison's artwork was featured in a series of commemorative postage stamps. I wish my dad had lived to witness that incredible honor.

***

Toward the end of the week, Rosemary, the county nurse, who had grown up across the street from our home, encouraged each of us – my mother, Joan, Sue, and me – to privately visit with Dad, giving him permission to die when he was ready.

Joan sat beside Dad talking about their mutual love of art. This bonded them from the time she was a child. What a precious gift she had given him by organizing his art show. And now, she was saying goodbye in a tender way, telling him that she would be okay.

When Sue left his bedside, she was emotional. She recalled that when she was a child, she frequently had a leg ache, and Dad had rubbed her leg. She told me that while she gave him permission to let go when he was ready, Dad started to rub her leg, sharing his love.

We each treasured that private time with him. When I assured him that we would care for Mom and each other, his face visibly changed. I'll never forget that. He had our permission to die. He was at peace.

As his doctor predicted, Dad died one week after his exhibit opened.

***

Midst gut-wrenching grief, Serena permitted Tim to let go when he was ready. She lovingly offered her dear husband permission to die, assuring him that she and Liam would be just fine.

I hoped that Tim felt at peace, hearing Serena's words.

24

On July 13, Tim had his last M-VASI infusion and his final medical oncology visit.

Hospice was ordered that day. Treatment ceased. Tim understood. The day was emotional for Tim and Serena. They shared this news with Liam, and although they didn't define "hospice," he understood.

July 13, 2022

Dear Serena and Liam,

Yesterday was so tough. Hearing the tumor was bigger. I just didn't want to believe it. Yesterday was a bad day. The doctor said I might just live for three days. I hope I will live for three months – maybe more.

I hope you will be able to get a photo of my tumor, Serena, so that Liam can understand it. But maybe you won't be able to.

Today I had an infusion – my last one. That was tough to say "good-bye" to everyone. I won't see them again.

Now, I am done with doctors. Done! No more.

I hope we will take a drive to Wisconsin in August. It would be so great to just see everything, to just relax, and laugh.

I have no pain. How could it grow? This is so bizarre. But I knew something wasn't right lately. At least I know now. And I am done with doctors.

And maybe the doctors are full of shit! Maybe I will live for weeks or months.

Love,

Either Tim misunderstood the doctor say that he may live for only three days or he mixed up "three days" and "three weeks," which is what his neuro-oncologist actually predicted.

In August 2021, when Tim was told he had 12-14 months to live, his immediate reply was that he intended to set a record. Throughout the months, that optimism never ceased, but it seemed to wane in July. Creeping into my conversation with Tim that day was his sense that something wasn't right.

Emotions hit a peak during that final oncology visit. Since Tim was diagnosed, his medical team had been there to educate, encourage, and support him. They were always honest with him. He knew that.

Still, he just didn't want to believe his life would soon end. After all, he had plans to spend time with Serena and Liam! He hoped to show them some of the sights he had loved while living in California. He wanted to join Liam on a golf course or tennis court. He wanted to run with Sammie. He wanted to surprise Serena with a special dinner at the top of the John Hancock building.

He wanted to visit his dad again, to learn more about his dad's full life, to hear how he and his mother had met. He wanted to laugh with Phil and Betty while they recalled funny escapades from their childhoods.

He wanted to see another Indy 500 with his pals, Scott, Drew, and Dave, or play another round of golf with Shaun.

***

How will I someday react to a final visit with my physician? I hope I will express gratitude. But if I still have a glimmer of hope, I might feel my doctor is giving up on me.

I can imagine, I too will find it difficult to say good-bye to my medical team who had been there through some tough times. But after enduring endless medicines, treatments, and medical appointments, I can imagine blurting out, "I'm done with doctors! Done! No more!" Tim was forceful when he said these words, and someday, I might be too.

25

The days of July were a blur for Serena. Monday blended into Tuesday, then into Wednesday and Thursday. She had stopped working on July 12 when Tim had his final MRI. She had no choice. She had to be with Tim nonstop.

Serena's dad, Chuck, and sister, Laura, stayed with the family for weeks at a time, but Tim wouldn't let them do very much for him. He wanted Serena to do everything. He insisted on her help. She was exhausted.

Whenever Tim lashed out verbally, she recalled how irritable he became early in their marriage at the most insignificant things. Over the years, that lessened or perhaps Serena had become accustomed to it.

Since his diagnosis, his irritability had nearly vanished. Until this month, he was always cooperative, accepting, grateful, and appreciative. Serena marveled at the difference. Now, anger resurfaced easily and unexpectantly.

Serena knew that he wasn't able to explain what he was doing – or saying:

"Why are you talking to me!?" Tim *yelled* at Serena.

"I'm talking to you, because I love you, Tim," Serena replied.

"Oh."

Tim may have been aware of feeling different emotions, but he couldn't understand them. He realized he was doing dumb stuff, saying words he didn't mean, but he didn't know why.

Tim became teary for no apparent reason. He couldn't comprehend what had made him cry. Serena tried to comfort him. He rested his head on her shoulder as he wept.

Limitations in doing the most basic things became apparent. Serena had been helping Tim bathe, then she hurt herself, straining to lift him out of the tub. (He outweighed her by 70 pounds.) Taking a bath ended that day.

She assisted him while taking showers, but she worried about his balance while standing, so she said, "Tim, please sit down in the shower," pointing to the shower chair. He didn't know what to do; he couldn't understand. That was the last time he took a shower. Going forward, she sponge bathed him.

Since Tim's diagnosis, Serena had marveled at his coordination in walking up and down the stairs. Even though he occasionally used a cane in the living room and on walks, he didn't require assistance when using the stairs, but now, that changed.

The right side of his body had become considerably weaker.

One morning, Serena awoke to the sound of breaking glass. She hurried to the kitchen to see shattered glass on the floor. Tim didn't understand how these things happened. They just did.

Another morning, she watched as his right hand brushed over the top of their bedroom dresser, knocking objects onto the floor. He looked up, confused. *How did that happen?*

Then, Tim startled her while walking down the stairs, suddenly dropping to his knees. Serena feared for his safety.

"It's time that you no longer go upstairs to sleep, Tim," she said. "I don't want you to hurt yourself. The right side of your body just isn't working like it used to."

Tim glared at her, not wanting to accept that, but knowing she was right. Still, he couldn't bear to hear Serena tell him he could no longer go upstairs.

Tim's final night sleeping upstairs was on July 14. The next morning, Tim awoke feeling dizzy and disoriented. Serena felt some solace, knowing that she had made the right decision in limiting Tim's movement to the living room level.

Liam watched his dad become weaker each day. Like his dad, Liam had hoped this downward spiral would cease, but early in Tim's diagnosis, his mom had used the term "terminal," and he figured it out. He didn't have to consult a dictionary.

***

When the hospice nurse arrived to care for Tim, Serena was relieved to have help. Tim was guardedly appreciative, but when the nurse asked to wash him, Tim balked. He did *not* want her to see him naked.

 "Tim, accept the help," Serena said. "Please, Tim. Please."

Although he felt humiliated, he agreed without complaint.

The hospice chaplain talked privately with Serena while Tim was being washed. Serena wondered what the end might be like. Based on her experience, the chaplain told Serena to not be surprised if Tim's dying moment happens when Serena has stepped away from his bedside.

"That seems to happen a lot as loved ones die, Serena, and you mustn't feel bad, nor feel any guilt," she said.

***

Pastor Joe Morrow from Fourth Presbyterian visited Tim and his family in mid-July, shortly before Tim's decline became pronounced. They visited for a long time. Pastor Joe's calming voice provided comfort to the family. Serena shared with me some recollections of their conversation.

"How are you today, Tim?" Pastor Joe asked.

Tim talked about how he was feeling, emphasizing that he was grateful to have no pain. He praised Serena, saying that she was providing "perfect" care for him.

"What is death like?" Tim wondered. "What will happen to me after I die?"

"You will find peace," Pastor Joe said. "You will feel welcome in Heaven."

"I think it will be easier for me, but harder for Serena and Liam," Tim said, with sadness in his voice. "Do you think loved ones who have died will be there to greet me? I hope I will see my mother."

Pastor Joe replied to every question with comforting words. Liam listened to his dad's questions and the pastor's answers.

The pastor prayed with Serena, Tim, and Liam, and they thanked him for his visit. Before leaving, Pastor Joe asked whether they had made decisions for Tim's memorial service.

Tim and Serena had started preparing for his memorial service eleven months earlier, shortly after Tim's diagnosis. For Tim's peace of mind, they needed to arrange the details of the service well in advance.

They envisioned Fourth Presbyterian filled with beautiful music, but Tim didn't request specific musical selections. He and Serena agreed on the names of those who would be invited to offer remembrances and read the eulogy at his service.

He emphatically told Serena that members of his immediate family would not speak at his service; he wanted them sitting in the front pew, enjoying the entire service.

26

Serena and Sammie greeted me when I arrived on July 18. I was convinced that no one entered the Hartwell home unless Sammie permitted it. As we walked upstairs, Serena told me Tim was very weak.

A hospital bed had been installed in the living room that morning. As I walked toward Tim, I thought he might be asleep, but he gradually turned toward me. "How do you like my new bed?" he asked, smiling.

"It looks comfortable."

"Yes, it is – so much better than the couch." His voice was weak, but he tried to project.

I no longer took notes as we talked; it just didn't seem appropriate. He needed my full attention. He asked me to move from the side of his bed to the end of it, so that he could see me easily without having to turn his head.

I looked at the end table beside him. Notecards, magazines, and calendars cluttered the surface. And then, I noticed a book. "Are you reading a new book?" I asked, turning it over.

"Yeah, I've just started."

"Are you kidding me, Tim?" I blurted as I noted the title. "*Quantum Book on Physics for Dummies*? Really, Tim? Are you interested in physics?"

"Not really," he replied, somewhat shyly. "I thought I should learn something about it."

Both of us chuckled. Then we laughed together loudly – and that felt good. Tim had to brush a tear from his eyes.

When I had texted Serena to arrange my visit, she told me that Tim often became emotional, so I wasn't surprised by Tim's tears, but I hadn't expected to see tears of joy. Serena also warned me that Tim tires easily, so that my visit may need to be brief. Perhaps Tim didn't get the memo; he was in a talkative mood.

He didn't describe the first indication of his brain cancer on the golf course in Lake Geneva; he didn't mention having to stay awake during his brain surgery; he didn't talk about doctors or hospitals. He didn't rave about his love for baseball. He didn't complain about his favorite Chicago teams.

He wanted me to know how wonderfully Serena was caring for him, how much fun it was to have Liam home during summer vacation. With a twinkle in his eyes, he asked whether I knew that Sammie was the best dog in the world. I assured him that I did.

Tim was excited to tell me that his childhood friend, Drew, had flown from Florida to Chicago a week earlier, his first visit since Thanksgiving. Prior to his visit, Serena had given Drew a sense of Tim's condition. She warned him that Tim's demeanor had changed, that he sometimes became angry or unpredictable. Days later, she texted Drew that he had just four to six weeks left.

When Drew arrived, his good friend was different. His face looked puffy, he spoke more softly, he was even more difficult to understand – but Tim's smile was the same. They greeted each other warmly.

Tim enjoyed telling me about the memories that Drew shared.

Drew reminded Tim how competitive he had always been. Shooting hoops, playing pool, throwing darts, it didn't matter – Tim was determined to win.

They had fun during sixth grade when they played for different teams in the same league. Drew was on the Phillies while Tim was on the Braves. Drew praised Tim, remembering his great arm, his talent as a left-handed hitter, and his intelligent instincts on the field. Tim smiled at the compliment.

Drew recalled their trip to play golf in Arizona. They were on the golf course at 8 a.m. As Drew prepared to tee off on the par-three second hole, he realized he would be looking directly into the sun, so he asked Tim to spot his ball. Drew's drive sounded great. He looked over at Tim for an indication of where his ball had landed. Tim wasn't paying attention. He was on one knee, tying his shoe, unaware that Drew's ball had dropped into the hole!

"I told you to watch it!" he yelled while Tim finished tying his shoe. "A hole in one – and you missed it!"

"Do you remember that day, Tim, my hole-in-one?" asked Drew. Tim didn't, but Drew guessed that Tim very likely remembered how HE had played that day.

27

My next visit was on July 29. Serena opened the door, and just stood there, looking drained of energy. She told me that her dad and sister were staying with her, then reminded me that Tim was now under hospice care every other day. I gently hugged her before heading upstairs. Sammie led the way.

I expected Tim to be asleep or at least resting but he was not. He greeted me from his bed, although I could tell that turning toward me was difficult. I again stood at the end of the bed so that Tim could see me easily.

"You were right, Tom," he said. "That physics book was dumb. Really stupid! It's gone."

"I'm not surprised."

"I have a new book over there, a book about Charles Schultz and his comic strips." He pointed to his bed stand.

"That's a better choice," I replied.

"I also have a new clock!" he announced. "Do you see it?"

After looking around, I didn't see it. With his left hand, Tim pointed up. Serena had added another large clock, projected on the ceiling above his bed. Now, Tim could delight in adding to his fascination with numbers.

"I can't move my right hand anymore," Tim said. "Not my right leg either. It's so strange – the right side of my body isn't a part of my body anymore."

"I'm so sorry, Tim. That must be tough."

"No. It's okay," he said, "but I can't get out of bed anymore, and that stinks."

I was stunned how matter-of-factly Tim described his new limitations. Since his diagnosis, he had been realistic – hopeful, but realistic. He told me about how polite and helpful the hospice aides were, and he was grateful that Serena had some help.

"I'm just so lucky. Liam doesn't have school, so he's home. Serena stopped working, so she's here. And of course, my pal, Sammie is always here." Sammie looked up at Tim.

"What's new with you?" He sounded almost jovial.

"We had a big family reunion in Missouri last week," I answered. "More than 100 people for four days. It's my mother's family, the Kretzschmars. Folks came from all over the United States and even New Zealand."

"That's huge," he said. "Do you do this every year?"

"No," I chuckled, "It takes a lot of planning, so we meet every four years. We started meeting in the 1970s. My Uncle Mart organized the first reunions."

"Do you always meet in – where was it?"

"Missouri. No, we meet wherever we can find a camp that will hold us. We'll be in Black Mountain, North Carolina, in four years." As soon as I said this, I regretted it, knowing that Tim could not think about four years from now, perhaps not even four weeks.

I changed the topic.

"Have you had any visitors lately?"

"Yes. Phil and my dad come a lot, and sometimes, Rose comes too. I think visiting me is hard on my dad, but I can tell that he really wants to spend time with me. I love him. It's tough for Phil and Rose too, but I'm doing okay. Everyone really helps me."

"Shaun stopped by a while ago," Tim added. "He makes me feel better even when I feel sorry for myself. He always cracks me up. Serena reminded me that he calls me 'Mr. Cranky Pants' sometimes."

"One time, Shaun teased me, saying that Serena would probably end up with a handsome quarterback," Tim said. Tim had told me several times that he never liked being teased as a kid or as an adult. Somehow, Shaun's teasing was funny, even endearing. They had that kind of a relationship.

"It's good to have Serena's dad here," said Tim. "He really helps us. We talk about business, but I know I'm hard to understand. I still try to read the *Kiplinger Report*." Tim was becoming weary.

"We've really had good conversations, Tom," Tim said. "Thanks for visiting me so many times."

"You're welcome, but I've enjoyed every minute. I've learned so much from you, Tim. I treasure all the conversations we've had. I will visit again next week."

"I love you so much, Tom."

"I love you too, Tim. You're my forever friend." We shook hands.

***

Serena walked with me downstairs. She mentioned how valuable her dad and sister had been during the past several months. Without their mother's presence, Laura had stepped into a maternal role at a time when Serena was overwhelmed.

She talked openly about her mother. Mother and daughter had always enjoyed a loving relationship, so Serena was surprised when her mom didn't offer to visit when Tim was diagnosed.

"My mom's absence deeply saddened me, but I could not dwell on this, because I faced many other worries related to Tim's illness," Serena said.

***

I drove home in silence, thinking about Serena and the burden she shouldered facing the days ahead.
I thought of Liam and the love that enveloped him from his mom, from Laura, and from Serena's dad, his Pa-Paw. I thought of Tim's hopeful attitude.

Toward the end of my life, I hope that I too will be grateful, hopeful, and realistic, that I will appreciate all of the kindness shown to me by family and friends.

28

Early the next week, Serena texted me that Tim was talking less and less. I proposed that I visit him Monday morning, and Serena agreed.

Liam had helped his dad by making a small poster listing various TV selections including the Golf Channel, Sirius 33 (alternative rock from the '90s), and Simpsons on I-Pad. Instead of expending the effort to speak, Tim just pointed to the one he wanted.

Because he was having trouble swallowing, Serena crushed his pills. He slept a lot. Those around him were quiet, hoping that Tim would sleep as much as he wished.

Sammie's behavior changed. Sometimes, pets know. Typically, Sammie rushed into the house after a walk. Now, he hesitated every time before coming inside. When he did, he approached Tim's bed reluctantly.

One day, Liam and his mom watched Sammie saunter toward Tim's bed, around it to the other side, and then he sat, staring up at Tim. Just looking at Tim for a long time. Suddenly, Sammie bounded down the stairs and remained there.

****

On Monday I awoke early to allow time for an early-morning walk in the neighborhood before leaving for Chicago. I finished a mug of coffee, then filled our bird feeder. The sun was shining through cumulus clouds.

Before opening my garage door, I received a text from Serena saying that Tim couldn't have any visitors today. He was in too much pain. I replied that I understood.

****

Serena had taken Sammie for a walk at 8 a.m. When she returned home, she went upstairs to change her clothes. Almost immediately, Laura called to her, saying, "Tim needs you."

When she went downstairs, Tim looked uncomfortable in his bed. Covers were thrown aside. As she walked to his bed, Tim looked at her, crying out very clearly:

"It hurts! I'm dying!"

"Oh Tim!" Serena said, feeling helpless.

"Serena, help me! I'm dying."

She touched him lovingly, holding his hand.

Serena gave Tim liquid morphine to ease his pain. He became calm, then fell asleep. His breathing was shallow but steady. He slept off and on for hours.

Serena called Phil to tell him that Tim was weakening. By mid-afternoon Tim's dad, Phil, and Rose were beside Tim.

Serena talked with a friend on her cellphone, telling him that it wouldn't be too long. Without warning, Serena suddenly said, "Oh, I have to go. Something is happening." She ended the call and quickly went upstairs to get Liam.

As Serena and Liam joined Tim's father, Phil, Rose, her dad, and sister, Tim faded away.

The date was August 8.

Tim would have enjoyed the symmetry of the date – 8-8-22.

29

Jane and I were among the first to arrive at Fourth Presbyterian Church on Saturday, August 20, for Tim's memorial service. Organ music, played by John Sherer, was already filling the sanctuary.

We sat quietly, in awe of the majesty of the church and the strains of Johann Sebastian Bach's "Soul, Adorn Yourself With Gladness" and my favorite, "Sheep May Safely Graze."

Before leaving home, Jane had asked me whether I thought there would be a large gathering for Tim's farewell. I guessed that an intimate group of relatives and close friends would gather. As more and more people filled the pews, I realized I had guessed incorrectly.

Tim's family walked into the sanctuary from a side door, moving to the front pews. I watched Serena and Liam take their seats. I spotted Serena's dad, Chuck. Then, I easily identified Phil; he and Tim resembled each other.

Associate Pastor Nancy Benson-Nicol officiated at the service. Her voice was strong and clear; her manner was comforting. As the assembly sang "Amazing Grace," I enjoyed hearing someone behind us sing the bass part to the familiar hymn. The pastor read the Scripture, then led a unison reading of Psalm 23. Three of us moved toward the front of church, walking up several steps to our seats near the dais where we would offer our remembrances.

Tim's friend from Florida, Drew Nielsen, spoke about Tim's optimism throughout his illness. Tim believed life was a blessing, and he never blamed God for his illness. He intended to maximize every day he had left, and Drew admired Tim's attitude. Drew's humor capturing Tim's habit of over-analyzing, whether on the golf course or selecting an engagement ring, tickled all who heard him speak. Tim had left quite an impression on his childhood friend.

Shaun O'Leary emphasized Tim's love for Serena and Liam, his kind and gentle ways. He had met Tim while in his first job out of residency at Evanston Northwestern Healthcare. His colleagues admired the empathy Tim had shown their patients in his role as practice manager. He and Tim played golf together. They attended sporting events including a Bears game where Tim had found some seats at a great price, seats so high they could see all the O'Hare flight patterns. Shaun's reflection concluded by saying when he is dying, he hopes to have the same grace that Tim had.

When it was my turn to speak, I described my unexpected, rich friendship with Tim which grew as we conversed over 12 months. I relayed his deep love for Serena and his hopes for Liam. I admired his optimistic attitude, and marveled at the phrase I heard Tim speak during every visit – "I am so lucky."

All three of us became emotional as we spoke. Losing Tim had that kind of an impact on others.

Scott Dickson didn't just read Tim's eulogy. He enhanced the events of Tim's life with interesting anecdotes, emphasizing how Tim made those around him feel good. He called Serena "a rock" for Tim during the past year. Scott admired Tim's sense of wonder. As much as he enjoyed sharing experiences with his friend, he received even more pleasure from watching Tim's eyes sparkle with every new experience. Beginning in 1989, when Tim landed at LAX on his first flight, Scott's life was enriched by Tim's friendship.

Before the pastor's commendation and blessing, the congregation recited "The Lord's Prayer" then sang the majestic hymn, "How Great Thou Art." Tim would have approved.

***

The reception following the service was lovely. A long receiving line extended through the large room. Serena looked emotionally drained, but she greeted everyone with warmth and appreciation for coming. I was pleased that she and Jane could finally meet.

While in line, I visited with Shaun O'Leary, Tim's longtime friend and golfing buddy. As a neurosurgeon, he had been so helpful to Serena during the entire year she cared for Tim.

I had hoped to talk with Tim's best friends, Drew Nielsen and Scott Dickson, but I never spotted them during the reception. I had hoped to meet his Indy 500 partner, Dave Farlee, but didn't.

I appreciated the opportunity to meet Tim's siblings, Betty and Phil, as well as their father. From my conversations with Tim, I felt I already knew them. Losing the youngest member of their family had to be so difficult.

Jane and I left the reception with Serena's dad, Chuck, who was, as always, a gentleman.

***

I was anxious to give Serena and Liam the gift from Tim – the 39 letters he lovingly left for them – but Jane convinced me that they needed time to grieve following the service. I waited patiently for more than a month before I drove to the Hartwell home in Chicago.

30

The days following the service were tough for Liam, but, according to his mother, his good friend, Kenny, was there for him.

A month after Tim died, school began. Although Liam looked forward to seeing his friends again, he was reserved. He missed his dad every day.

On the first day of sixth grade, Liam wrote a poem for an assignment, then stuffed it in his backpack.

His mother didn't find it until she cleaned out the backpack on June 7, 2023, his last day of sixth grade. Serena said she was "wrecked" when she read it.

Grapevine
By Liam Hartwell
6th grade 2022-2023

Cranes tower over like giraffes
Bulldozers crush buildings
It looks like the sky is falling
All I hear is Crunch! Crunch! Crunch!
Four flocks of flying fish I see in the distance
They dig up the earth and make a giant hole
The only thing left is one light pole
As it falls my heart breaks
My whole world crushed into pieces
Everything is still all right
Everything is still fine
Because there is still my beloved grapevine

31

I visited Serena and Liam on October 5, 2022, two months after Tim died. Serena looked refreshed as she opened the door for me, with Sammie by her side, of course.

Gone were the lines of stress from Serena's face. She and Liam seemed to be working through their grief. They smiled easily as we visited.

I was pleased to see that Chuck remained with his daughter and grandson, helping in big and small ways. He had been their constant support from the time Tim entered hospice through the fall, helping Liam adjust to the beginning of the school year.

Serena lovingly showed her appreciation for my visits with Tim and my remembrance at the memorial service. Liam was polite as usual. He smiled as I hugged Sammie.

Before leaving, I gave Serena and Liam a present of fruit and sweets to enjoy. Hidden beneath was Jane's beautifully wrapped present – the black binder of precious letters from Tim. I left quietly as they began to unwrap the present.

****

Serena wrote to me the following morning, saying in part:

*"Liam was very tearful last night, missing Tim.
I often feel the same way, looking for something
tangible to make me feel better.
This compilation of letters is so special, and
the cards really got me.
This book means more than you know."*

Epilogue

Fall moved into winter, then Christmas and New Year's 2023. On Saturday, January 21, I was excited to visit Serena and Liam again. Sammie and Liam greeted me. I told Liam that he looked like he had grown, and he smiled in return.

*****

I had a burning question for Serena: "Did Tim slip in revealing our secret? Did he tell you about the surprise book of letters?"

Serena acknowledged Tim's vague recollection that he and Tom had planned a surprise, but she had no idea what it was. In time, she had forgotten his comment. She was completely surprised to open the present of the black binder. They read all 39 letters immediately.

***

No seagulls have landed on Serena's shoulder yet, but when she hears seagulls squawking, she thinks of Tim. She figures that he's trying to get her attention. She now appreciates the beauty of seagulls as they soar gracefully over Lake Michigan.

Several days after Tim died, she walked to her car. Two seagulls flew overhead making noise until she bothered to look up. Then, they stopped.

In mid-August 2023, when she and Liam arrived at their favorite Lake Michigan beach, she watched Liam take off running on the sand. Amazingly, there beside Liam, was a seagull running beside him.

*****

A Babe Ruth baseball card hasn't yet been found for Liam, but he's still hopeful. Interestingly, Liam has decided to start saving football cards.

*****

Serena waited months before she was able to separate Tim's ashes into three containers as he had desired.

Ashes were scattered from a walking bridge in Prosper into a river below. Tim's dad, Phil, and Rose joined Serena, and Liam. This was where the ashes of Tim's mother had been scattered.

In July 2023, ashes were scattered a mile out from the Lake Michigan beach where the Hartwell family enjoyed walking.

Serena and Liam scattered Tim's ashes that autumn at the Field of Dreams in Iowa, a place that reflected Tim's love of baseball and his deep love for his family. A warm summer breeze greeted them as Liam, Serena, and Sammie raced around the bases several times. Serena had just turned 50.

*****

Liam was 5'3" when his dad became ill. Now, in January 2024, Liam is very close to 5'8". His childhood doctor was correct; he's going to be tall.

Some nights, as Liam is trying to fall asleep, he smiles, thinking of spending time with his dad, walking to a field at DePaul where his dad throws the football while he runs play patterns that his dad has *meticulously* designed. He imagines watching his dad grin while hitting a wiffle ball a mile.

He thought of his dad in mid-September 2023 while sitting with his mom, imagining the huge grin on his dad's face as Cubs infielders Mark Grace and Shawon Dunston were inducted into the team's Hall of Fame.

*****

Serena received a telephone call from Liam's Language and Literature teacher at school. The teacher had assigned her class to conduct research based on a book, then prepare a "Ted Talk" to present to the class about their topic.

Liam chose the topic of "Glioblastoma." Ms. Wilcox called Serena to tell her that Liam's classmates were entranced as they listened to Liam's very personal story about the disease that took his dad's life.

*****

Loved ones who have lost someone dear to them occasionally experience something that reminds them of the person they lost. Liam and Serena are no exception.

Days after the funeral, Serena, Liam and Serena's dad were somewhat startled to hear the refrigerator make the sound of a heartbeat – similar to a sonogram – just once.

Nearly a month after Tim died, on September 3, 2022, just before falling asleep, Liam saw a clear image of his dad's face at the foot of his bed surrounded by a triangle and five figures of people.

On many occasions but not all, when Serena enters Tim's closet, the light flickers.

In September 2023, when Serena and Liam visited Tim's dad, they were surprised to look out his third-floor window to see a hummingbird hover. No flower boxes are anywhere nearby.

Finally, just before Christmas 2023, Serena dreamed of Tim. She and some friends were enjoying a boat ride toward an island. As they entered an inlet, Serena was in awe as she saw a beautiful open area filled with tropical flowers and trees. She walked up a hill and sat in a swing with the friends, but when they left her alone, there was Tim, looking young and healthy. He smiled at her, his face surrounded by a glow, a glow of comfort and relief. Perhaps Tim had come to visit.

*****

A photo of Tim is displayed on a small easel in my office, a daily reminder of my friend and the lessons he shared with me.

I think of that day in August 2021 when I received his unexpected call. I think of the first time he greeted me in his home, flashing that familiar Hartwell smile. I think about his delight in leaving a surprise gift for Serena and Liam, his precious letters. I think about how lucky I have been to know Tim Hartwell.

Author's Note

Several people who were aware of my visits with Tim asked whether the idea for writing a book came to me while I was visiting him. The answer is no.

I didn't mention the possibility of writing a book to Serena until January, 2023—six months after Tim died. Had I thought of writing a book while Tim was alive, I would have asked very different questions.

Acknowledgments

Writing a first book is daunting, but I've enjoyed the entire experience. Standing beside me through the journey has been my wife, Jane. I've been so fortunate to have her understanding, love, and support as well as her on-target editing suggestions.

Even before I wrote my first sentence, three cousins and several former students unknowingly encouraged me simply by publishing their own books.

Several members of Tim's family, as well as a few friends, agreed to be interviewed.

A team of beta readers provided me with direction, criticism, and valuable ideas as they read the earliest portions of my manuscript. Many thanks to Sue Hildebrand, Mike Joyce, Jamie Mulvenna, Richard Nelson, and Jared Olson. Assistance in helping me understand the publishing world was offered by Julie Kendrick, Lizzie Nelson, and Jess Wright. In addition, Susan Cahalan helped me deal with the unique challenges of writing a nonfiction book.

Three editors offered invaluable assistance. They are a treasure.

Jill and Dave Stewart dove into proofreading and editing my book, offering constructive suggestions, pertinent observations, and insightful questions. (Thanks, Dave, for gently reminding me that the ruins in Pompeii are not in Greece but instead in Italy!) In addition, I'm grateful for their help in suggesting marketing strategies to increase the book's visibility.

Executive editor Nancy Arnesen spent countless hours in a deep dive of editing, asking the tough questions, focusing on developmental editing, providing her style of brutal honesty, and helping me confront and overcome unexpected hurdles, while always encouraging me.

Popular author and artist Rod Vick was invaluable as I neared the finish line, preparing to publish. His assistance in formatting, design of the book cover, and calm demeanor even when I felt harried were just what I needed.

Finally, Tim's wife and son opened their home and hearts to me throughout the past year. Their love and encouragement have been absolutely amazing.

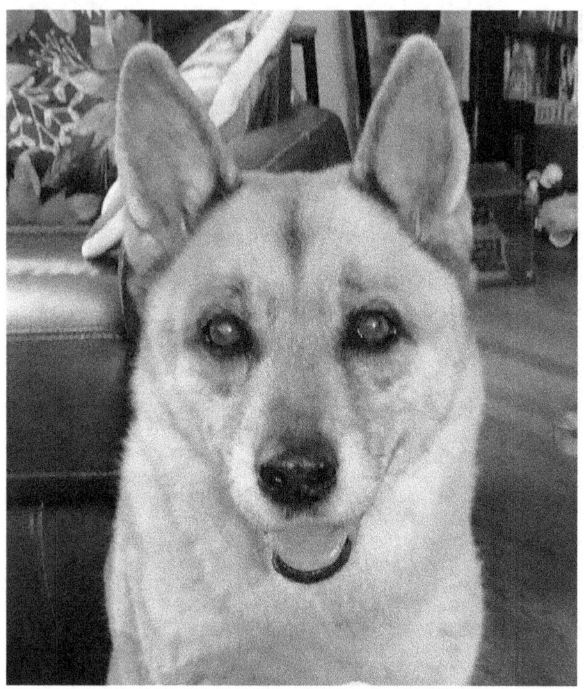

Sammie

Throughout Tim's final year of life, Sammie was a comfort and joy for the family. He continues to provide that same comfort now to Serena and Liam.

Random reader reactions to Unexpected Gifts

In recent travels, including to Louisville for the 2023 Sweet Adelines International convention, I approached random strangers asking them a question: "Are you an avid reader?" If they replied affirmatively, I invited them to read and react to my manuscript. I also invited a few others.

"This story is a poignant reminder to us that life is fleeting and that living and dying with grace is the gift we give those we leave behind." (Susan Stevens, Carson, WA – middle school English teacher)

"A very touching encounter and a great reminder that God puts us in the right place at the right time more often than we may know. A thought-provoking yet refreshing book." (Duane Warriner, Perry, NY – packaging technician)

"Unexpected Gifts is an enthralling read. A story of determination and friendship that attains that rare but precious level of agape. May it inspire the same kind of devotion in everyone who reads this extraordinary tale." (Tracy Hulett, Carol Stream, IL – strategy and leadership)

"Beautiful story that follows a tragic medical condition and the courage and fortitude exhibited by those most affected. This story should bring comfort to anyone facing similar circumstances." (Park Bierbower, Chambersburg, PA – human services in state government)

"If you want help in having awkward discussions with seriously ill family or friends, you will find this book full of helpful, real-life information. I wanted to stay with the story until its conclusion." (Marigail Jones, Point Arena, CA – retired registered nurse

"As someone who has walked a very similar journey, I found an emotionally satisfying story that should comfort all who have faced or will face the cancer journey alone." (M. Christine Enoch-Rogers, Bristol, IL – realtor and legal assistant)

"A beautiful story that reminds us to cherish the people who God placed in our lives. A story that calls us to share in each other's journey. A story that inspires us to face the end of our own journey with grace and love." (Lynnette Lewis, Madison, AL – retired bus driver)

"Can the time spent with a friend make a lasting difference? This is the touching story of how one man's love and faith did just that. Memories are made of this." (Kathy Bierbower, Chambersburg, PA – small business owner and community volunteer)

"Toftey's story not only conveys an appreciation to the reader for his friend, Tim, and for the strength of his remarkable wife and young son through this unimaginably difficult time—he also shows how any one of us can make a difference in someone's final journey through the small, simple act of helping Tim leave behind a precious gift for his loved ones. It's an engaging book on a sad subject that somehow manages to be, when all is said and done, uplifting." (Kristy Aserlind, Livingston, MT – ski instructor and fly fishing guide)

About the cover art

My dad, Adolph (Ade) Toftey, was the editor and publisher of the *Cook County News Herald,* the weekly newspaper in Grand Marais, Minnesota. The youngest of 11 children, he was the only one born in America. Ade was a fisherman, avid rockhound, historian, writer, bass in the church choir, self-taught violinist, fluent in Norwegian.

But Ade's passion was art. When he was 15 years old – after begging for two years – he convinced his parents to pay $25 for a two-year correspondence course in political cartooning. Becoming a cartoonist never happened, but he pursued his love of art at Carleton College, Northfield, MN, graduating in 1926 as its first male art major.

The Depression dampened his interest in art, but in 1937 he married Bertha, and she encouraged him to return to painting. And that he did. Until his death in 1991, Ade painted more than 300 water colors and oils using the landscape of the rugged north shore of Lake Superior as his canvas. His paintings are found in private collections, businesses, universities, and museums throughout the country and also in Norway, his ancestral home.

The cover featuring a large oil painting he titled "Gulls Over Ice Floes" (1980), is owned by my sister and her husband, Sue and Dave Hildebrand.

About the Author

After teaching English and journalism, working in communications, corporate relations, and market research, Tom Toftey has added "author" to his list of careers with this book. He has taught writing, spoken at conferences, and written articles for magazines and newspapers.

A native of Grand Marais, Minnesota, Tom and his wife, Jane, are loyal Midwesterners, now living in Winfield, Illinois. They are the proud parents of two children and the grandparents of five.

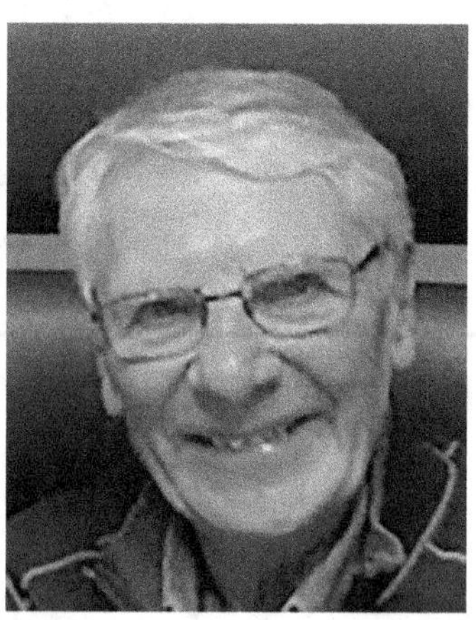